Journey Into Life

High/Scope Educational Research Foundation, Ypsilanti, Michigan

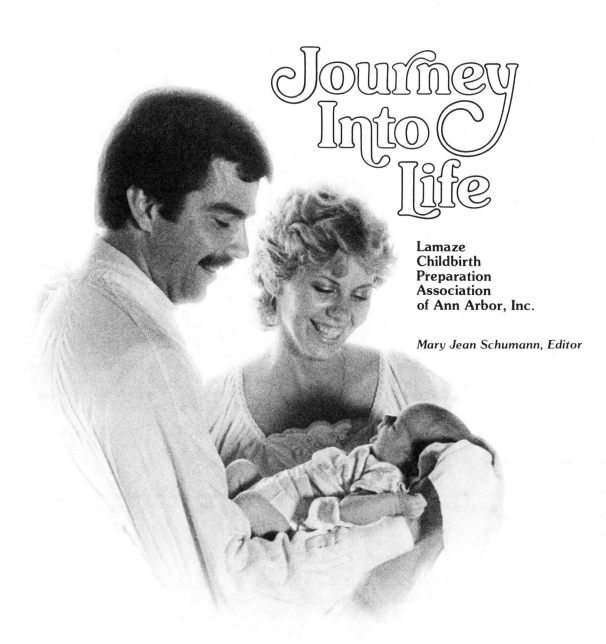

Journey Into Life

**Lamaze
Childbirth
Preparation
Association
of Ann Arbor, Inc.**

Mary Jean Schumann, Editor

The High/Scope Press

Published by
THE HIGH/SCOPE PRESS
High/Scope Educational Research Foundation
600 North River Street
Ypsilanti, Michigan 48197
(313) 485-2000

Gary Easter, Photographer
Linda Eckel, Designer
Mary Hohmann, Press Editor
Michael McGowan, Illustrator

Photographs courtesy of the Catherine McAuley Health Center, Ann Arbor, Michigan: pages 5, 6, 62 (right), 125, 129, 135, 150, 154. Photographs courtesy of the Lamaze Childbirth Preparation Association of Ann Arbor, Inc.: pages 105, 118 (right).

Library of Congress Cataloging in Publication Data

Journey into life.

   Bibliography: p.
   Includes index.
   1. Pregnancy. 2. Childbirth. 3. Natural childbirth.
4. Infants (Newborn)—Care and hygiene. I. Schumann,
Mary Jean. II. Lamaze Childbirth Preparation Association
of Ann Arbor.
RG525.J68   1983   618.2   83-13010

ISBN 0-931114-22-5

Printed in the United States of America.

Contents

5018717

Acknowledgments

The authors of the third edition of this text are instructors for the Lamaze Childbirth Preparation Association of Ann Arbor, Inc. They include Phyllis Cant, Ruth Ann Corwin, Sue Gillespie, Marsha Goodhart, Mary Lou Greenfield, Cathy Griffin, Cathy Haskins, Marie Heys, Kathy Krajewski, Linda Lampman, Carole Mayer, Fran Mayes, Sue McMillan, Barbara Okonkwo, Joan Paskewitz, Nancy Rogers, Mary Jean Schumann, Pat Van Bonn, and Carol Ziemiecki. Other contributors are Roberta Crosby, Mary Schuman, Mary Ann Stark, Jan Valentine, and Kathy Welch. A special thanks to Beth Gall for her expertise in developing Chapter 9, to Pat Rutowski and Dan McMurtrie, MD, for their careful reading and validation of the text, and to Ruth Ann Corwin for her assistance in the writing and editing process. Thanks also to the many people who contributed to the earlier editions, especially Trish Booth who served as their editor.

Mary Jean Schumann
Editor

Journey Into Life

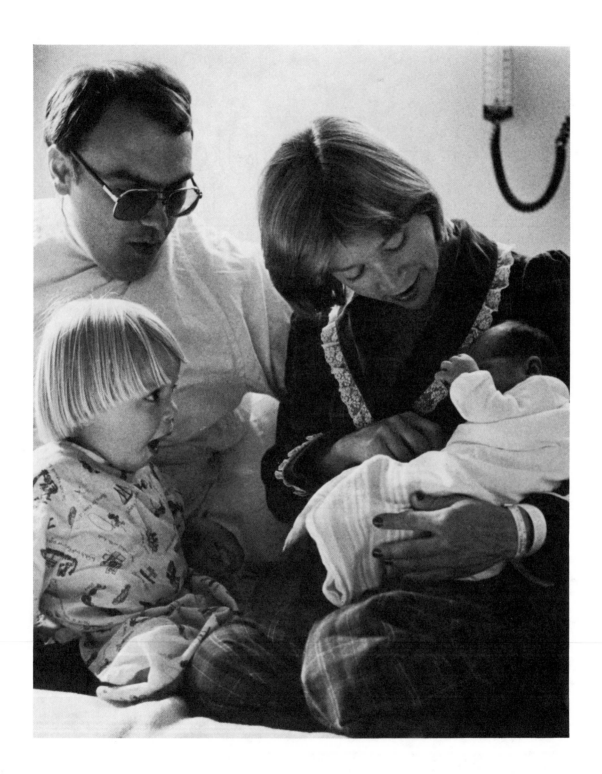

CHAPTER 1

Prepared Childbirth: Principles and Options

The origin of the Lamaze method

At the 1950 World Congress of Gynecology in Paris, French physician Fernand Lamaze met a group of Russian psychologists who claimed they could make childbirth painless by applying Pavlov's principles of conditioned response to the childbirth process. Dr. Lamaze was so impressed by their presentation that he went to Russia to study their methods and to see for himself women giving birth without pain. Upon returning to France, he founded a program called "Childbirth Without Pain." In addition to incorporating the Russian methods, the "Lamaze method" introduced breathing techniques devised by Dr. Lamaze.

Today the Lamaze method of childbirth is practiced throughout the world—in the United States, Europe, South America, Africa, and parts of Asia.

Psychoprophylaxis: Using your mind to dull or prevent pain

Three factors affect pain in childbirth:

- Physiological pain is caused by signals the contracting uterus sends to the brain.
- Fear of the unknown (What is happening to my body? What next? When will this end?) exaggerates your perception of the amount of pain you are feeling.
- Body tension resulting from fear contributes to discomfort.

The Lamaze method prepares you for childbirth through psychoprophylaxis (psycho = mind, prophylaxis = prevention)—using your mind to prevent the pain caused by psychological fear and body tension, and to dull physical pain. Lamaze classes teach you to alleviate or dull your perception of childbirth pain.

Overcoming physiological pain

The brain receives pain signals from the contracting uterus. The brain also controls breathing. Contractions are involuntary processes and cannot be controlled. Breathing, however, can be controlled. When a woman in labor controls her breathing as a learned response to the beginning of a contraction, her brain cannot concentrate on both the breathing pattern and the pain signals from the uterus. Therefore, as a result of her concentration on breathing, her perception of pain is peripheral and more easily ignored. The patterns of breathing taught in Lamaze classes require great concentration, thereby increasing their psychoprophylactic effectiveness.

Conquering the fear of the unknown

Thorough discussions of labor, delivery, and hospital procedures calm many of a woman's pre-delivery doubts and fears. Knowing what to expect gives her a feeling of confidence and eases the tensions of her partner as well.

Releasing body tension

Uterine contractions are involuntary, but many other muscle groups can be relaxed at will. The Lamaze method teaches special techniques of "conscious relaxation." The woman and her partner practice these techniques so they can easily recognize body tension and act effectively to reduce tension in voluntary muscles.

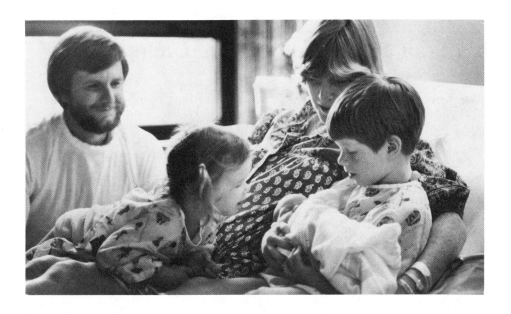

Family-centered birth in a hospital setting

Because complications of the birth process have an unfortunate way of occurring very quickly when least expected, our association does not advocate or encourage home deliveries. Instead, our association is working to provide a more natural, family-centered birth experience within the hospital setting. Specifically, we work together with hospital staff to bring about procedures that will permit

- Parents or partners and, in some cases, siblings to be together throughout labor, delivery, and recovery.

- Parents and baby and, in some cases, siblings to spend time together immediately after delivery as long as the conditions of the mother and the baby permit. This time together fosters closeness and the development of bonds between the baby and family members.

- Rooming-in so that parents get to know their baby before leaving the hospital.

- Sibling visits to lessen the trauma of separation, establish the older child's relationship with the baby, and help decrease the older child's resentment and feelings of being left out.

- Grandparent visits to extend support to new parents.

Birth options available in the United States

There are as many ways to experience childbirth as there are women. As you consider your options, you will want to determine your own feelings about

- Where you would like labor and birth to occur
- In what type of atmosphere you would feel most comfortable
- How much time you would prefer to spend in the hospital before going home
- The amount of contact you would like to have with your baby in the hospital
- The people you want to be present during labor and birth

The traditional hospital setting
Traditionally, the woman and her partner labor in a specially designated, hospital labor room until early in the second stage of labor when they are transferred to a room specially equipped for delivery. Usually delivery is followed by a one- or two-hour recuperation period in a recovery or private room, after which the woman is transferred to the postpartum (afterbirth) unit of the hospital. In many hospitals, only the labor partner

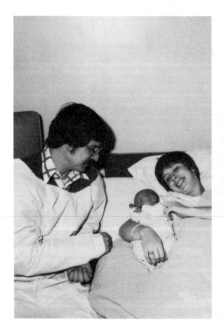
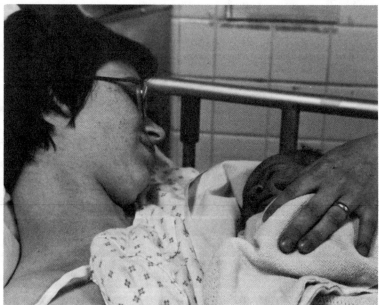

is allowed to observe the birth and spend the immediate recovery period with the mother and/or the baby. A baby's time with parents before going to the nursery varies from 10 to 60 minutes.

When a birth might be complicated by the need for forceps, a breech presentation, twins, or a cesarean delivery, most women and health care providers opt for the safety of a hospital delivery room, where staff and equipment are readily available.

The labor room

Sometimes the woman and her partner labor and give birth in a labor room within the hospital's labor and delivery unit. Recuperation may occur in the labor or the recovery room of the hospital. The baby may stay with the mother, father, and, occasionally, other family members for up to 60 minutes, or may never be separated to go to the nursery. Sometimes labor-room birth is followed by a short stay on the post-partum floor and then discharge as early as four to six hours after birth. However, the mother has the option of staying at the hospital for two or three days if she wishes.

A woman whose labor is progressing typically and who does not anticipate complications may choose this option, although some health care providers prefer that a woman experiencing her first birth does so in a hospital delivery room.

The birthing room, suite, or center

Some hospitals have birthing rooms, or suites, furnished with a double bed, easy chairs, and bath and kitchen facilities, where the woman and her partner labor and give birth. While the atmosphere is more relaxed and casual than it is in a traditional labor room, emergency hospital equipment is close by so that hospital staff can give medical help immediately, if necessary. In some hospitals, the woman completes her postpartum stay in this room. Because of their home-like atmosphere, birthing rooms and suites can accommodate siblings during labor, birth, and recovery. The baby may stay with the mother until discharge, and early discharges are fairly common.

A woman wishing to give birth in a birthing room or suite must have a preliminary prenatal exam, describe her health history to hospital staff, and fulfill hospital criteria to ensure an uncomplicated birth.

A birthing center can be located either within or close to a hospital. The birthing center permits a woman to give birth in a home-like atmosphere where emergency care is only moments away. The whole family may be present at the birth, the baby is not separated from the family, and early discharges are common.

A woman choosing to give birth in a birthing center is carefully screened prenatally in an attempt to avoid complications that might endanger her or her baby.

Home birth Occasionally a woman and her partner prefer to labor and give birth at home attended by a midwife and/or a physician. A woman considering the home-birth option must take into account the availability of back-up emergency care and the philosophy of the health care provider who will assist in the birth.

Making the choice Choosing the type of birth experience most suited to you is a matter for you and your partner, together with your health care provider, to assess. Your own health will play a vital role in the birth process wherever it occurs.

Selecting health care for yourself

Your continuing health care is vitally important to you and your child throughout your pregnancy and after your baby's birth. During your pregnancy your health can be responsibly managed by a family practice physician, a certified nurse midwife, or an obstetrician (a specialist in the care of pregnant women). The services of these professionals are available in either private offices or public clinics.

To obtain names of appropriate health care providers, you may want to take the recommendation of a friend, relative, or physician; contact the hospital of your choice to find out which professionals deliver babies there; or seek recommendations from health-care-oriented consumer groups.

Once you have a list of health care providers, call each one and do some preliminary screening by phone conversations with staff members. After this screening, arrange appointments for visits with two or three persons you are still considering.

During this first visit, note the atmosphere of the office, note how the person's staff relate to you, and decide if you respect the person enough to cooperate with recommendations for your care. In addition, you may want to ask some of the following questions:

- What are the health care provider's specific qualifications and how significant are they to your care? How medically competent is the health care provider?

- Is this a solo or group practice? Who will deliver your baby if the health care provider is not available at the time of your delivery? In a group practice, how often would you see the other health care providers? Do group members share a similar philosophy of prenatal health care and childbirth, or do they represent a range of opinions and options?

- How are the fees handled and how much are they? Ask for specific amounts for prenatal care, vaginal birth, cesarean birth, postpartum follow-up, and six-week postpartum checkup. Does the health care provider accept the fees established by your insurance agency?

- What are the views of the health care provider regarding prepared childbirth, management of uncomplicated labor and birth, the father's participation during vaginal and cesarean birth? Does the hospital share the same views?

- How does the health care provider respond to questions? Is enough information conveyed to enable you to follow recommendations? Is there an organized approach to patient education?

- What is the role of nursing personnel? What interaction do they have with you?

- How receptive are the health care provider and staff to family members accompanying you on prenatal visits?

- How responsive are the staff to your phone calls?

- What services does the health care provider offer after the birth of your baby (circumcision, routine gynecologic care, well-baby care)?

In your search for a health care provider, you need to be aware that some physicians employ an obstetric nurse clinician. This person is a registered nurse, frequently holding BS or MS degrees, who has completed additional studies in the needs and care of childbearing women. An obstetric nurse clinician works with physicians and other members of the health care team to assess the physical, emotional, and social health of clients and to provide periodic prenatal exams, nutrition counseling, and information about pregnancy, birth, and postpartum adjustment. The obstetric nurse clinician may be more accessible than the physician to respond to your concerns by telephone. After your child's birth, the obstetric nurse clinician may make daily hospital rounds to discuss your concerns and provide discharge information and teaching.

If you have a low risk of developing difficulties during pregnancy and delivery, you may wish to consider the services of a certified nurse mid-wife (CNM).* A CNM follows you through your pregnancy; delivers your baby in a hospital with a back-up physician on call; and provides post-partum follow-up, birth control information, and routine gynecologic care. A CNM usually has more time than a physician has to spend with you both prenatally and during labor. Because her caseload is usually small, a CNM may spend the entire labor with you plus one or two hours after delivery. If you go home within 24 hours, a CNM may also make

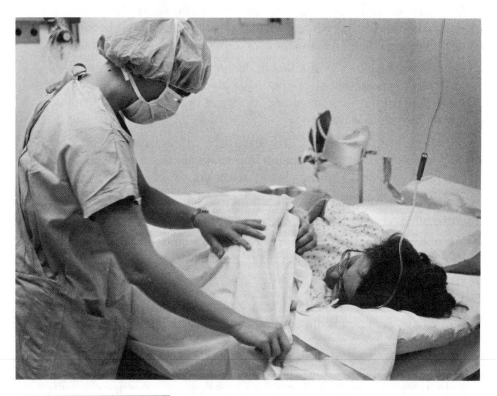

* A certified nurse midwife is a registered nurse with additional training in pregnancy, childbirth, and postpartum care. A CNM possesses evidence of certification according to the requirements of the American College of Nurse Midwives. State legislation passed in 1978 permits the practice of nurse midwifery in Michigan. You should check to see if legislation permits the practice of nurse midwifery in your state.

a visit to your home one or two days later. Fees vary depending on insurance coverage.

Women who are not good candidates for care by a CNM include women with a history of chronic illness like diabetes, heart disease, or renal disease, or with a history of difficulty with previous pregnancies, including a previous cesarean delivery, repeated spontaneous abortions, or premature births.

Whether you choose a family practice physician, an obstetrician, or a certified nurse midwife, you can expect that during each prenatal visit, your health care provider will inform you about your health and well-being and your baby's health and well-being. These visits are also your opportunity to discuss any questions and concerns you may have about your pregnancy, labor, and delivery. Following is a checklist you may want to use to remind yourself of issues to discuss with your health care provider during your prenatal visits. These issues are reviewed in detail throughout this book.

Things to review with your health care provider about pregnancy, labor, and delivery

Pregnancy

- ☐ Are there dietary recommendations? Will I need vitamin or iron supplements?
- ☐ Are there restrictions on medications, cigarettes, alcohol, caffeine, drugs?
- ☐ What exercise restrictions should I follow?
- ☐ Are there any restrictions on working during pregnancy?

Labor

- ☐ Who fills out hospital preadmission forms? How are they obtained?
- ☐ Should I attend childbirth classes?
- ☐ Can I eat during labor?
- ☐ When my membranes rupture, what do I do?
- ☐ Under what circumstances should I call my health care provider?
- ☐ When should I go to the hospital/birthing center?
- ☐ When will the health care provider arrive at hospital/birthing center?
- ☐ Under what circumstances might induction of labor occur?
- ☐ Is the use of fetal monitors routine?
- ☐ Is the use of IV (intravenous injection) routine?
- ☐ What medications will be available to me during labor and why?
- ☐ What is the possibility of cesarean delivery?

Birth

- ☐ Who may be with me during birth?
- ☐ May my partner be present if and when anesthesia is used?
- ☐ Must I give birth in a delivery room or can I do it in a birthing room?
- ☐ In what positions may I give birth—side-lying, semi-sitting, kneeling on all fours, squatting, lying on back?
- ☐ Might forceps be used? When?
- ☐ Are episiotomies routine?
- ☐ Is photography, videotaping, or recording allowed?
- ☐ Is viewing the birth possible? By whom?
- ☐ What special arrangements can be made—dimmed lights, water bath?
- ☐ When can the baby be held, breast fed?
- ☐ What are choices for eye medication for baby? Can it be delayed?
- ☐ How long can my family remain together?

Hospital stay

- ☐ What types of rooms are available—private, semi-private, ward?
- ☐ Is rooming-in available—24-hour, daytime, on demand?
- ☐ What are visiting hours for father, siblings, relatives, friends?
- ☐ What will be my baby's feeding schedule?
- ☐ What teaching occurs in hospital/birthing center—breast feeding, bottle feeding, bathing, diapering, care of episiotomy?
- ☐ When do I have to decide about circumcision?

Discharge

- ☐ What is the minimum hospital/birthing center stay for vaginal birth? For cesarean birth?
- ☐ When can my baby be discharged?
- ☐ When can swimming, running, or a regular exercise program be resumed?
- ☐ When should I become concerned about vaginal discharge—lochia, bleeding?
- ☐ What are birth control options?
- ☐ When can intercourse be resumed?
- ☐ Whom can I call about breast feeding concerns?
- ☐ What local support groups are available?

Additional considerations if you are planning a cesarean birth

Preoperative procedures

☐ Will ultrasound be used to assess gestational age?
☐ Will I have a trial of labor (chance to deliver vaginally by monitoring progress of labor)?
☐ When will my delivery be scheduled?
☐ When will I enter hospital—morning of cesarean or night before?
☐ Will I have medication for sleeping the night before surgery?
☐ Will I need an enema?

Anesthesia

☐ Should I make a pre-delivery appointment with anesthesiologist?
☐ May my partner be present during administration?
☐ Is pain medication available after birth? How is it given?
☐ Will I be awake or asleep during birth?

Birth

☐ What type of incision will be made?
☐ How will the incision be closed? Stitches or staples?
☐ May my partner announce baby's sex?
☐ May my partner hold baby? Will my hands be free to touch?
☐ Will baby remain in delivery room for exam?
☐ May my partner remain with me and go to nursery?

Recovery room

☐ May my family be together?
☐ May I breast feed in the recovery room?

Hospital stay

☐ Will I have a cesarean mother for roommate?
☐ Will my baby stay with me if I have a low-grade, postoperative fever?
☐ How soon may I return to a solid diet?
☐ When will catheter and IV be removed?

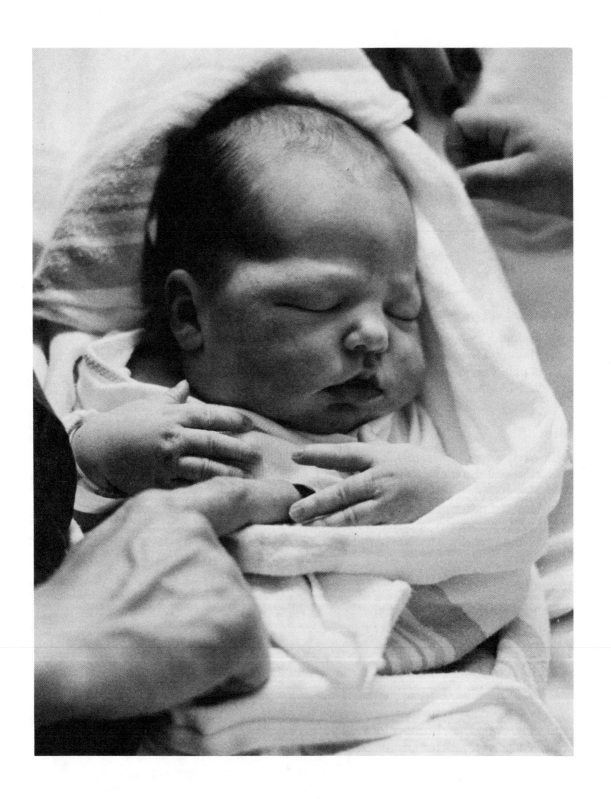

CHAPTER 2

Maternal Nutrition and Fetal Development

Nutrition: When you eat well, you help your baby grow

Nutrition during pregnancy has not always been regarded as a critically important issue. For much of this century, for example, doctors and scientists assumed that babies could draw all the nourishment they needed before birth from their mothers regardless of what their mothers ate. We know now that pregnant women do not instinctively eat to meet their own nutritional needs and the nutritional needs of their unborn children. Therefore, during the past decade, nutritionists and doctors have established specific nutritional guidelines for expectant mothers.

Pregnant women gain weight because of the physiological changes they experience as their babies grow. The current recommendation for weight gain during pregnancy is 24 to 30 pounds. Underweight women are encouraged to gain weight. Overweight women also need to gain weight as their babies grow and develop and should, therefore, avoid dieting during pregnancy. Although a 27-pound weight gain is an average gain of three or four pounds a month, many women find they gain weight in spurts—five or more pounds during a month when the baby is growing rapidly and one or two pounds during another month when the baby's growth is more gradual.

Weight gain

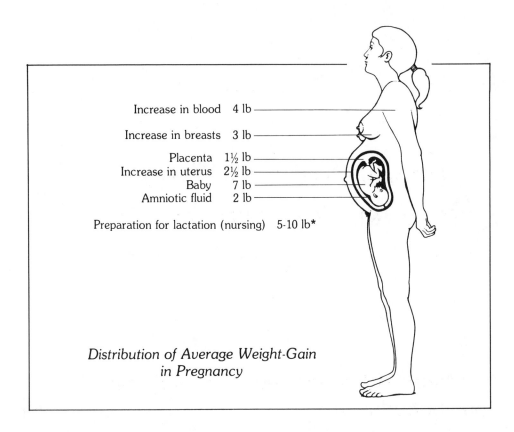

Increase in blood   4 lb
Increase in breasts   3 lb
Placenta   1½ lb
Increase in uterus   2½ lb
Baby   7 lb
Amniotic fluid   2 lb

Preparation for lactation (nursing)   5-10 lb*

*Distribution of Average Weight-Gain
in Pregnancy*

Salt Your total fluid increase during pregnancy is between six and eight quarts. Therefore, you need salt to maintain fluid balance and to allow for adequate blood expansion. Use iodized salt, and do not restrict your salt intake unless your health care provider specifically advises you to do so.

Prenatal vitamin and mineral supplements Since it may be difficult for pregnant women to meet their requirements for iron and folic acid through diet alone, health care providers frequently recommend or prescribe supplements. Your requirement for folic acid doubles during pregnancy. Your body's need for iron increases markedly as a result of a two-quart blood increase. Even though pregnant women can meet other vitamin and mineral requirements by eating properly, health care providers often prescribe prenatal vitamins. Such supplements, however, are no substitute for a well-balanced diet.

A well-balanced diet Pregnant women who each day eat a variety of foods from the "basic four" food groups—milk and milk products, protein foods, fruits and

---

* An increase in general body fat occurs providing an "emergency reserve" for a lactating mother, should she, for any reason, need to temporarily reduce or halt her own nourishment.

vegetables, and breads and cereals—can meet their own and their babies' nutritional needs for everything except iron and folic acid.

Basic diet for pregnancy and nursing

Food group	Minimum daily requirement	Food sources
Milk and milk products	4 cups for pregnancy 5 cups for nursing	Whole milk, low-fat milk, skim milk, buttermilk Milk products equivalent to 1 cup of milk in protein and calcium content: Cheese (1½ ounces) Cottage cheese (1¼ cups) Plain yogurt (1 cup)
Protein foods	6-8 ounces for pregnancy 8-10 ounces for nursing	Beef, pork, lamb, fish, veal, poultry Substitutes for 1 ounce of meat: Egg (1) Peanut butter (2 tbsp.) Dried beans (½ cup cooked) Tofu (½ cup)
Fruits and vegetables	4 servings (½ cup each) for pregnancy and nursing	All vegetables and fruits
Breads and cereals	4 servings (½ cup or 1 ounce each) for pregnancy 5 servings for nursing	Cereals, breads, crackers, rice, pasta
Fluids	8 cups during pregnancy 10 cups during nursing	Beverages including: Milk Fruit juices (unsweetened) Vegetable juices Water

Teen diets   If you are under 18 years old and pregnant, you will want to give extra attention to your diet. Because your own body is still developing, you have greater nutritional needs than an older woman who is fully developed. Make it a point to talk to your health care provider about your dietary needs and requirements during pregnancy.

Vegetarian diets   Vegetarians who eat eggs and milk products while they are pregnant and breast feeding can meet their nutritional needs, while those who add chicken and fish to their diets substantially improve their nutritional intake. Women on a vegetarian diet can increase protein quality by eating specific combinations of vegetable proteins during the same meal:

- Corn with beans
- Rice with beans
- Breads and cereals with beans
- Peanuts with wheat, oats, corn, or rice
- Garbanzo beans with sesame seeds
- Tofu with sesame seeds
- Soy flour with wheat, corn, or rye

If you are a vegetarian and pregnant, review your diet with your health care provider to make sure you are meeting your increased need for calcium and vitamin B-12.

Eating patterns   During your pregnancy, eating smaller meals or snacks more frequently throughout the day may decrease the discomfort of fullness and heartburn and allow you to avoid feeling faint from hunger or sluggish from eating too much.

Substances and situations to avoid   Although you cannot control all the factors influencing your health and the health of your unborn baby, there are certain substances you can avoid. The degree to which your baby can be affected by these substances is not always known. However, the advantages of avoiding them for nine months far outweigh any inconvenience this may cause.

   Most medications and unprescribed drugs you take pass from your circulatory system, through the placental* barrier, and into the baby's

* The placenta, connected to the baby by the umbilical cord, is the structure through which the baby receives nourishment from the mother.

blood. Therefore, it is important for you to check with your health care provider before taking any medication. Evidence links alcohol consumption to birth defects. Although there is uncertainty as to the amount of alcohol it takes to undermine fetal development, many health care providers recommend limited or no consumption of alcohol during pregnancy. The caffeine you drink also reaches your baby. Since the effects of caffeine on babies are not altogether known, health care providers recommend that you limit the amount of caffeine-containing products in your diet.

As nicotine from cigarette smoking passes from your bloodstream to your baby's, it interferes with the efficiency of the placenta, decreasing the amounts of nutrients and oxygen that reach the baby. The more a pregnant woman smokes, the greater the risks she is taking with her own health and the health of her baby. Nicotine in breast milk may also be harmful to babies. During the first year of life, babies whose parents smoke have higher rates of pneumonia and bronchitis than do babies of non-smokers. Older children whose parents smoke have twice as many respiratory infections as do older children of non-smokers. Fortunately, studies have shown that it is never too late in pregnancy to stop smoking and receive positive effects from doing so. If you smoke, it is wise to cut down or stop smoking during pregnancy. Since this will probably not be easy, you may wish to enlist the encouragement and support of others to help you.

Parasite eggs living in cat litter and raw meat cause toxoplasmosis, a disease harmless to adults but potentially dangerous to a baby in utero (in the uterus). You can avoid these parasites by eating only well-cooked meat and staying away from cat feces. If you are a confirmed cat lover, wear rubber gloves when it is your turn to empty the litter box, or better yet, have someone else empty the litter box while you are pregnant.

Unnecessary x-rays may be harmful to your baby, along with fumes from cars, paint, household cleaners, some glues, and pesticides. Since these toxic substances can enter your blood through your lungs and skin, work outside or in well-ventilated areas if you must be near these products. Wear gloves to protect your skin, and limit your exposure as much as possible.

Ultrasound is thought to be safe and is preferable to the use of x-rays for some purposes. However, since studies of the long-term effects of ultrasound on pregnant women and babies are still being conducted, it may be wise to limit ultrasound to diagnostic use.

Fetal development: How your baby grows inside you

What you eat influences both your health and comfort during pregnancy and the growth and development of your baby from the time your baby is conceived. Your well-balanced diet promotes your baby's growth. The following are highlights of your baby's growth and development prior to birth. (See Chapter 3 for a more complete discussion of conception.)

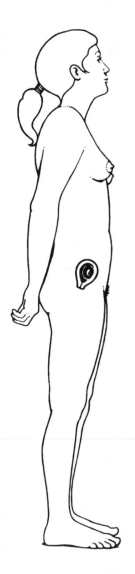

End of the eighth week

Day of conception. After intercourse, the mother's egg and the father's sperm join, and fertilization occurs.

Days 13-21. The fertilized egg travels from the mother's ovary, down her Fallopian tube, and into her uterus.

Day 22. The fertilized egg attaches itself to the uterus. The placenta begins to form.

Sixth week. The backbone, spinal canal, and head are forming. The embryo (fertilized egg) is 1/12 inch long and 1/6 inch wide. The heart begins to beat.

Seventh week. The chest and abdomen are completely formed. The eyes are apparent. The embryo is now approximately 1 inch long.

Eighth week. The face, arms, legs, hands, and feet are partially formed. The embryo weighs 1/15 ounce and is now called a fetus. Its slight movements are not yet detectable by the mother. Facial features are forming, including the palate and the jaw. The mother's uterus is still hidden inside her pelvis.

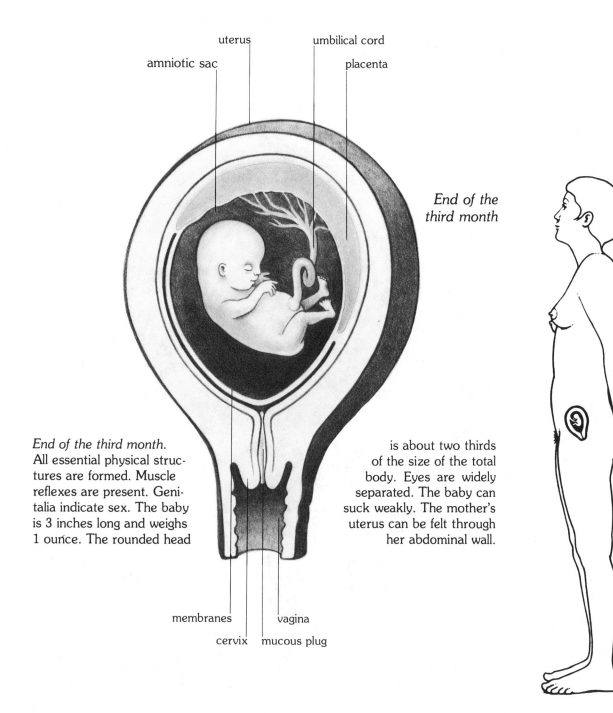

uterus

amniotic sac

umbilical cord

placenta

End of the third month

End of the third month. All essential physical structures are formed. Muscle reflexes are present. Genitalia indicate sex. The baby is 3 inches long and weighs 1 ounce. The rounded head

is about two thirds of the size of the total body. Eyes are widely separated. The baby can suck weakly. The mother's uterus can be felt through her abdominal wall.

membranes

vagina

cervix

mucous plug

Maternal Nutrition and Fetal Development   21

*End of the
fourth month*

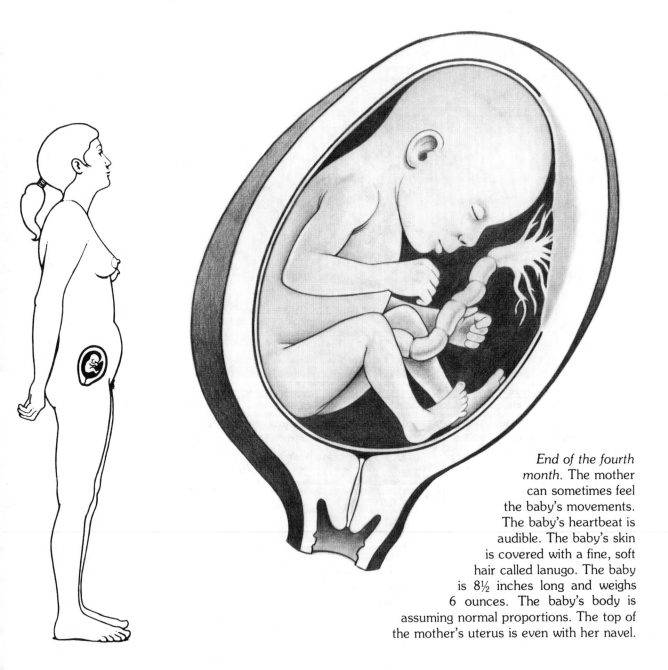

*End of the fourth
month.* The mother
can sometimes feel
the baby's movements.
The baby's heartbeat is
audible. The baby's skin
is covered with a fine, soft
hair called lanugo. The baby
is 8½ inches long and weighs
6 ounces. The baby's body is
assuming normal proportions. The top of
the mother's uterus is even with her navel.

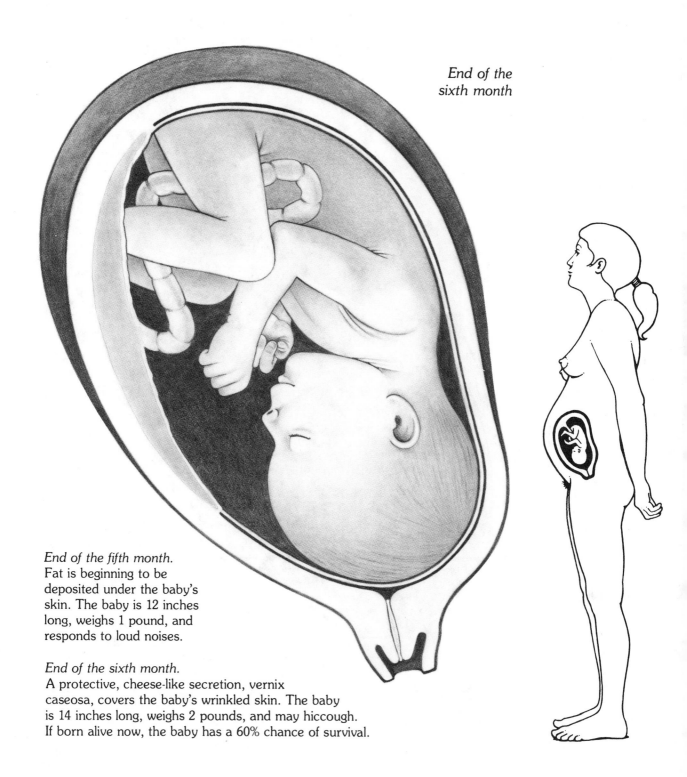

End of the sixth month

End of the fifth month.
Fat is beginning to be deposited under the baby's skin. The baby is 12 inches long, weighs 1 pound, and responds to loud noises.

End of the sixth month.
A protective, cheese-like secretion, vernix caseosa, covers the baby's wrinkled skin. The baby is 14 inches long, weighs 2 pounds, and may hiccough. If born alive now, the baby has a 60% chance of survival.

Maternal Nutrition and Fetal Development   23

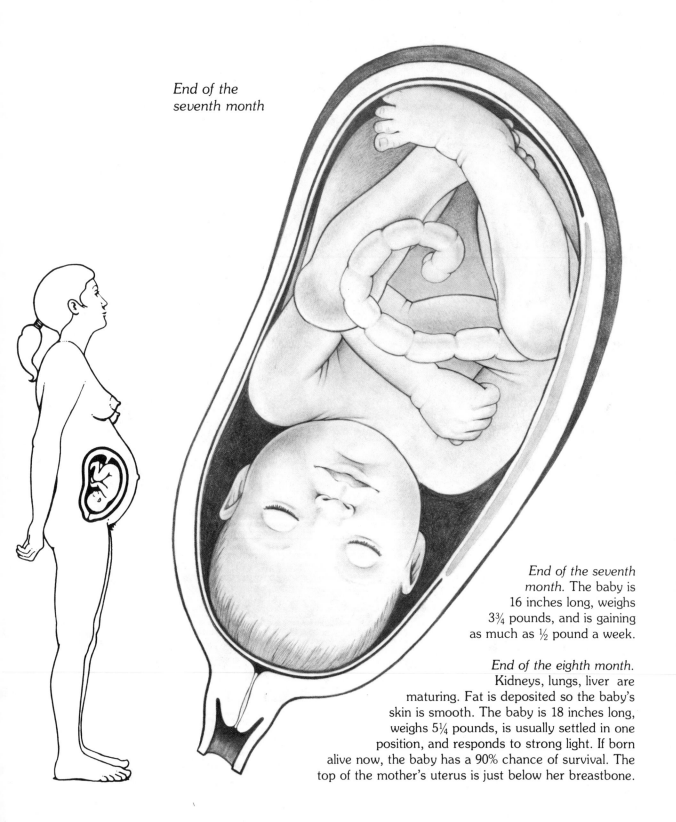

*End of the
seventh month*

*End of the seventh
month.* The baby is
16 inches long, weighs
3¾ pounds, and is gaining
as much as ½ pound a week.

End of the eighth month.
Kidneys, lungs, liver are
maturing. Fat is deposited so the baby's
skin is smooth. The baby is 18 inches long,
weighs 5¼ pounds, is usually settled in one
position, and responds to strong light. If born
alive now, the baby has a 90% chance of survival. The
top of the mother's uterus is just below her breastbone.

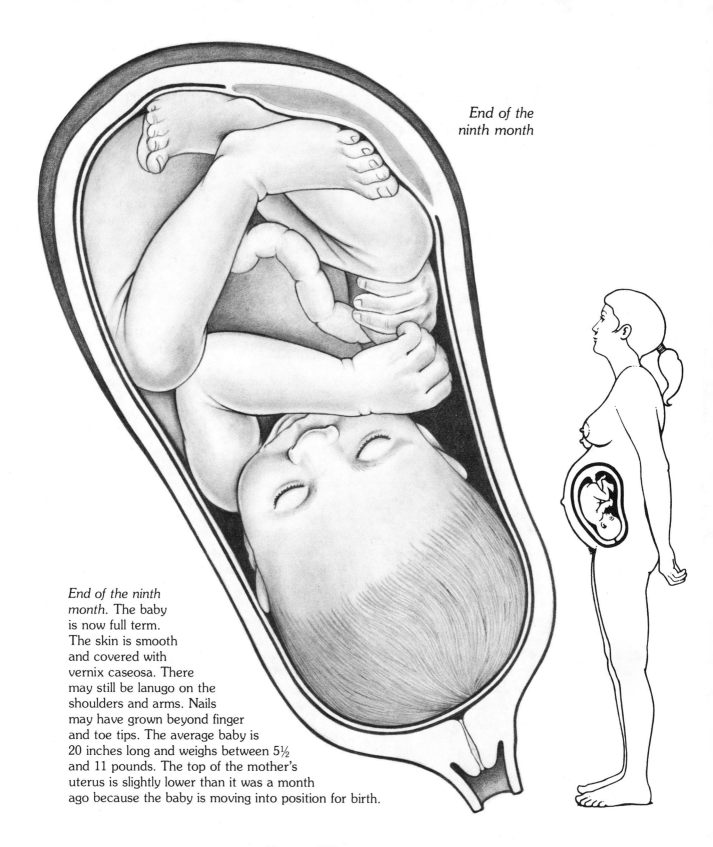

End of the ninth month

End of the ninth month. The baby is now full term. The skin is smooth and covered with vernix caseosa. There may still be lanugo on the shoulders and arms. Nails may have grown beyond finger and toe tips. The average baby is 20 inches long and weighs between 5½ and 11 pounds. The top of the mother's uterus is slightly lower than it was a month ago because the baby is moving into position for birth.

Ways of assessing your baby's growth and health before birth

In addition to the routine urine and blood-pressure tests you receive at every monthly prenatal visit, there are other tests your health care provider may wish to do during your pregnancy to assess the health and maturity of your baby. Few women undergo all of these tests and many women never need any of them. They are described here, however, so that should you need them, you can discuss them with your health care provider.

An ultrasound scan One possible test (called an echogram or ultrasound scan) produces a picture of the baby in the uterus. High frequency sound waves pass through the mother's abdomen and bounce off the baby's solid structures, into a transducer (microphone) placed on the mother's abdomen. These echoes are converted into an electronic image (scan) of the baby which is displayed on a small television screen. This image is photographed and interpreted by a radiologist. A health care provider may request a scan in order to confirm pregnancy, establish the estimated date of delivery, assess fetal maturity (age and stage of development but not lung maturity), determine the position of the baby and the placenta, verify the presence of more than one baby, or detect congenital abnormalities (physical problems that may be present at birth).

The procedure for an ultrasound scan is painless. Before your appointment, drink the prescribed amount of water and refrain from urinating for approximately an hour before the scan is scheduled so your bladder is full and your uterus is pushed upward. This makes both organs more visible on the scan. At your appointment, you will undress, put on a hospital gown, and lie on your back under the scanner. A gel will be spread on your abdomen to help conduct the sound waves. The ultrasound transducer will then be passed over your abdomen in different directions. When your baby's image appears on the screen, it will probably look like a confusing array of dark and light dots. Ask your health care provider to explain the image by pointing out different parts of your baby. This test may last from ten minutes to an hour, depending on the baby's activity.

Amniocentesis A sample of amniotic fluid may be taken from the mother's uterus to diagnose certain congenital and hereditary abnormalities and to determine fetal lung maturity. Prior to amniocentesis, ultrasound is frequently used to locate the position of the placenta and the baby. Once a safe position for needle insertion has been located, the mother is usually given a local anesthetic. A needle is inserted through the mother's abdominal wall into the amniotic sac (the protective "bag of waters" surrounding the baby), and about half an ounce of amniotic fluid is withdrawn. The amniotic fluid, containing cells from the baby's skin and other organs, is tested in a laboratory for chromosomal abnormalities. Then the fluid, minus the cells, is tested for alpha-feto protein (AFP), indicating certain congenital anomalies. Amniocentesis to determine abnormalities is done around the sixteenth week. Occasionally amniocentesis is done later in pregnancy to test fetal maturity.

It is possible to test the mother's blood for alpha-feto protein which, if present in abnormally high levels, can signify possible defects in the baby's nervous system. This test is done only if it is warranted by family history or maternal history. Since AFP levels in pregnant women double every five weeks in the fourth, fifth, and sixth months of pregnancy, AFP screening is usually done before the eighteenth week, when AFP levels tend to be low. If test results are abnormal, screening may be repeated for verification, or an ultrasound scan and/or amniocentesis may be recommended.

Maternal serum AFP screening

Another test measures the concentration of the hormone estriol in the mother's urine. As pregnancy advances, the level of estriol normally increases in a predictable way. When a pregnant woman develops high blood-sugar (gestational diabetes), her estriol level sometimes does not increase or may decrease. (See Chapter 3 for a discussion of gestational diabetes.) Her health care provider may need to investigate the situation. Since the level of estriol may be affected by factors not associated with pregnancy, this test is not entirely foolproof, and repeat estriol determinations may be necessary for more complete and reliable results. The test for estriol is most often done on urine collected over a 24-hour period, but it may also be done on urine collected immediately upon rising in the morning.

Estriol determination

Sometimes it is desirable to record the baby's movements during a specified time period each day. Although most babies become less active near term (before birth), a marked decrease in fetal movement may be a warning signal that should be evaluated. A mother can do this test at home at a convenient time by recording the number of fetal movements she feels during the specified time period. Periodically the mother's health

A fetal movement chart

care provider reviews the chart, evaluates the amount of activity, and, if necessary, recommends a non-stress test.

Maternal daily record of fetal movement

Your Name_____ Health Care Provider_____

DATE		Total:	AM		Total:	PM	Day
Gross + 3 sec.							
Short 1 - 3 sec.							
Very Short — 1 sec.							
(Rhythmic)							
	Last Meal:	Smoking:		Last Meal:	Smoking:		
DATE		Total:	AM		Total:	PM	Day
Gross + 3 sec.							
Short 1 - 3 sec.							
Very Short — 1 sec.							
(Rhythmic)							
	Last Meal:	Smoking:		Last Meal:	Smoking:		

A non-stress test
Another kind of test records the pattern of the baby's heartbeat in response to movement. Often done to evaluate the health of an overdue baby, this test takes place at a hospital because it uses a fetal monitor. An external fetal monitor is attached to the mother's abdomen. When she feels her baby move she pushes a button which transfers a mark to a tape recording the baby's heart rate. Normally, a baby's heart rate increases when the baby moves. When the baby's heart rate accelerates, the baby is reactive and the test is positive. If the baby's heart rate does not increase with movement, the baby is non-reactive and further testing may be in order.

An oxytocin-challenge test
To determine if a non-reactive baby (and sometimes an overdue baby) is at risk and should be delivered, a stress test is sometimes performed. This test takes an hour and occurs in a hospital. The mother receives an intravenous infusion of oxytocin, a hormone that induces uterine contractions. During the contractions, the fetal monitor records the baby's heartbeat pattern. Usually, the baby's heart rate slows down with each contraction and returns to normal soon after the contraction ends. If this occurs, the baby is not under any particular stress. If, however, the baby's heart rate remains slow after the contractions end, the baby may be at risk, and your health care provider may decide that labor should be induced or that a cesarean delivery is necessary.

Sometimes it is necessary to determine whether the baby is getting enough oxygen during labor. Fetal blood sampling is done when the mother is in active labor, her cervix is dilated three centimeters or more, her membranes are ruptured, and the baby's head or buttocks are well down in the mother's pelvis. A small sample of blood is taken from the baby's head or buttocks. If the sample is normal, the baby is getting enough oxygen and no immediate action is necessary, although additional blood samples may be taken later on. If blood acidity is increasing, the baby is receiving less oxygen. If birth is imminent, labor is usually allowed to proceed. If not, a cesarean delivery may be necessary.

Fetal blood sampling

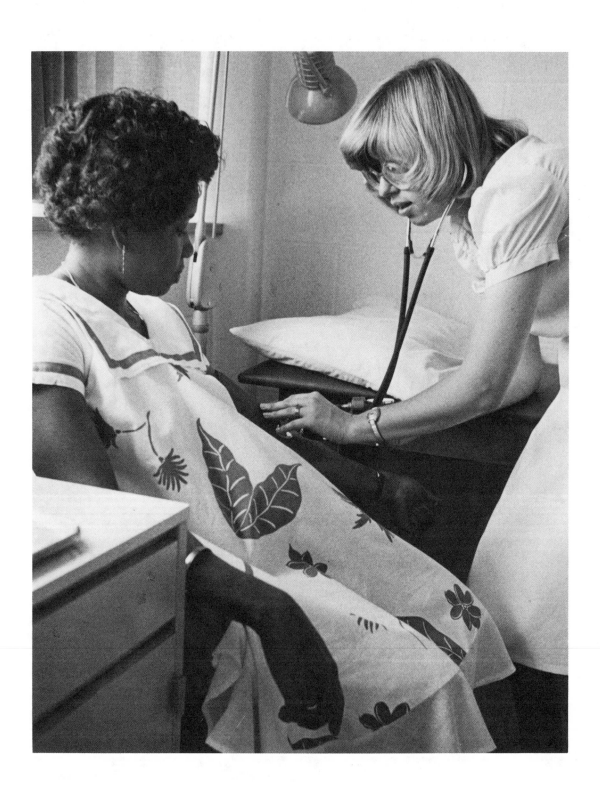

CHAPTER 3

Understanding Your Changing Body During Pregnancy

Conception: Pregnancy begins

To understand the childbirth process, a basic knowledge of the human reproductive organs is essential. Such knowledge improves communications with your health care provider and with your own children as you talk with them about "where babies come from."

Externally, male genitalia consist of the penis and the scrotum. The scrotum is a wrinkled bag of skin that houses the testes. The penis includes the urethra, a tube that carries urine and semen, and erectile tissue that, when filled with blood during sexual excitement, causes the penis to become erect. Internal male reproductive organs are the testes and a canal system. The testes manufacture sperm cells, which are transported to the urethra by the canal system.

Male anatomy

The external female genitalia include the vulva, the clitoris, the urethral opening, and the vaginal opening. The principal internal female reproductive organ is the uterus, a hollow, pear-shaped organ approximately two to four inches in length, widest at the top, or fundus, and narrowing to a thick, circular closing called the cervix. The cervix

Female anatomy

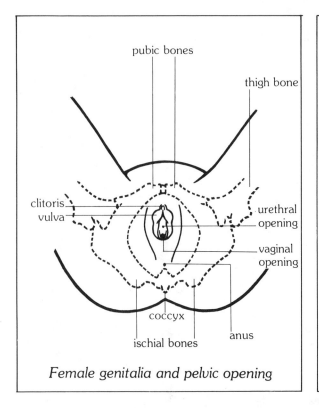

Female genitalia and pelvic opening

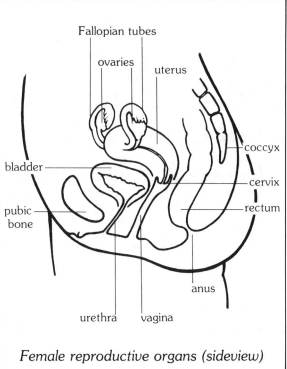

Female reproductive organs (sideview)

extends into the vagina, the passage connecting the internal and external reproductive organs. Extending from both sides of the uterus are the Fallopian tubes through which the ovum (egg) travels after it is released from the ovary once a month.

In relation to other pelvic organs, the uterus is tipped slightly forward, with the bladder directly below the uterus and the pubic bone directly in front of the bladder. Behind the uterus is the rectum and behind the rectum, the coccyx, or tailbone. Externally, the openings of the bladder, uterus, and rectum are, respectively, the urethra, the vagina, and the anus.

The rectum, uterus, and bladder are supported by muscles and ligaments (connecting tissues) in the bony pelvis, which includes the two ischia (hip bones) connected to the coccyx by the sacrum in the back, the pubic bones in front, and two ischial bones on which the body rests when sitting. Together, these bones form a protective basin for the reproductive organs. The size and spatial configuration of these bones are important because, to be delivered vaginally, the baby must be able to fit through the pelvis.

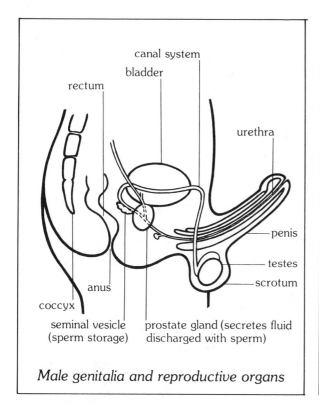

Male genitalia and reproductive organs

- rectum
- canal system
- bladder
- urethra
- penis
- testes
- scrotum
- anus
- coccyx
- seminal vesicle (sperm storage)
- prostate gland (secretes fluid discharged with sperm)

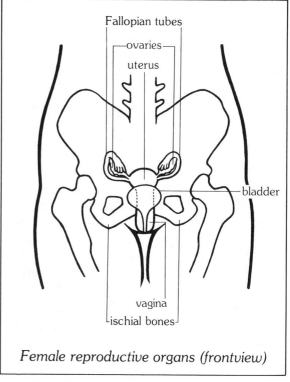

Female reproductive organs (frontview)

- Fallopian tubes
- ovaries
- uterus
- bladder
- vagina
- ischial bones

Conception

Approximately once a month one of the female's ovaries releases an ovum (egg) into one of her Fallopian tubes. If the egg is not fertilized by a male's sperm during intercourse, the egg travels through the Fallopian tube and into the uterus, from which it is discharged (along with the lining of the inner uterine walls) during menstruation. If the egg is fertilized by a male's sperm cell during intercourse, the fertilized egg travels through the Fallopian tube for several days, its cells already dividing and growing, and attaches itself to the uterine wall. Here the fertilized egg further divides into the embryo (the baby in its earliest stage of development), the placenta, and the amniotic sac. The placenta, a vascular organ through which the baby is nourished, is attached to the uterine wall and to the baby's umbilical cord. The umbilical cord contains one vein through which the mother passes oxygen and nourishment to the baby, and two arteries through which the baby passes carbon dioxide and wastes back to the mother. The mother's blood and the baby's blood generally do not mix, but both circulate through the placenta where substances diffuse from one's blood stream to the other's. Inside the placenta, the baby is enclosed in membranes that are filled with amniotic fluid in which the

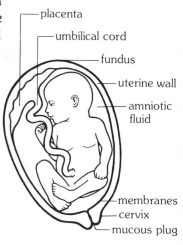

- placenta
- umbilical cord
- fundus
- uterine wall
- amniotic fluid
- membranes
- cervix
- mucous plug

baby floats, moves, and is cushioned from outside movement. As further protection, the small opening of the cervix fills with mucus and forms a plug which acts as a barrier against bacteria.

A new center of gravity: Posture for pregnancy

As your baby grows, taking up more room inside you, adding weight to the front of your body, and extending your abdomen, your center of gravity shifts forward. This shift can cause lower-back strain, but it does not have to if you maintain an awareness of your posture throughout pregnancy.

A normal adult spinal column has four curves—two relatively unchangeable primary curves, the thoracic and sacral curves, and two very moveable secondary curves, the cervical and lumbar curves (which maintain the balance necessary for upright posture).

The relatively unchangeable thoracic curve accommodates the heart, ribs, lungs, and sternum. The vertebrae in the sacral curve are fused together and therefore immoveable. It is the woman's moveable lumbar curve that is most affected during her pregnancy. To compensate for the forward shift of her center of gravity, a pregnant woman tends to thrust her chest out and shoulders back, which exaggerates the lumbar curve in the small of the back. Consequently, some pregnant women, to maintain balance, rely increasingly on their lower-back muscles and less and less on their abdominal muscles. This strains the lower back, causes backache, and diminishes needed abdominal muscle tone.

On the other hand, a pregnant woman who consciously practices good posture can avoid backache and strain. Abdominal muscle control is the key. Abdominal muscle control helps hold the abdomen in, preventing the center of gravity from shifting any further forward than it needs to. As you pull your abdominal muscles in, you also (1) bring your tailbone forward, decreasing the lumbar curve in the small of your back and (2) tip your pubic bones upward, giving increased support to your growing abdomen and enlisting the pelvic floor muscles in the support of the uterus from below.

Correct posture during pregnancy is a matter of concentrating on standing tall, holding in the abdomen, and tilting the pelvis forward and up. At first, it may require thought and effort to maintain this posture,

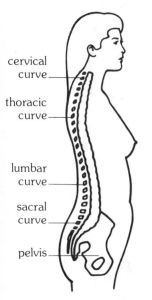

cervical curve

thoracic curve

lumbar curve

sacral curve

pelvis

cervical curve

thoracic curve

lumbar curve

sacral curve

pelvis

but once you get in the habit, you will look better, feel better, and tire less quickly.

The following exercises will help you maintain good posture and avoid backache during pregnancy because they are designed to condition the back, abdomen, and pelvic floor muscles. To prevent strain and fatigue, do these exercises slowly. Start by doing the exercises five times a day and try to include them in your normal daily routine.

Stand 12 inches from the wall with your feet about 12 inches apart. Bend your knees, place your hands on your knees, and lean your tailbone against the wall. Drop your head and shoulders forward, curling your back. Keeping your knees bent, uncurl your spine as you slowly tilt your pelvis so that your tailbone rolls away from the wall and the small of your back presses into the wall. When your back is flat against the wall, straighten your legs and bring your feet close to the wall. Take a deep breath to relax your shoulders and walk away standing tall, continuing to maintain the pelvic tilt.

The posture check

The posture check

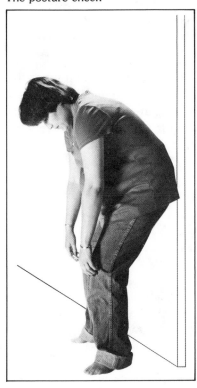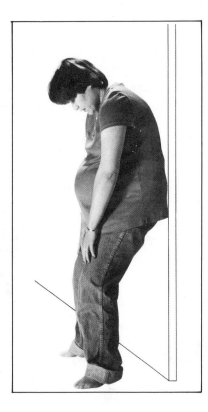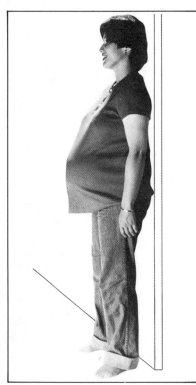

Back stretching This exercise promotes lower-back muscle flexibility needed for correct posture. Sit on the floor with your hands on your knees, your knees apart and flexed, and your feet flat on the floor. Inhale as you roll back, curving your spine into a "C" curve, with your shoulders rounded and pelvis tilted. Then exhale as you straighten your back and pull your body forward, keeping your back straight and your chest out. Lean forward from the hips. Your bent arms will be parallel to the floor. Work toward bringing your ears in line with your knees. Repeat.

Back stretching

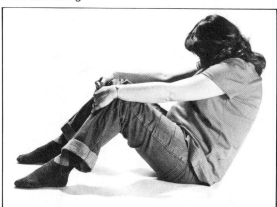 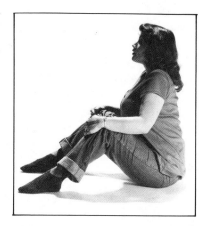

Wide stride stretches This exercise promotes leg and lower-back flexibility. Sit on the floor with your legs straight and comfortably separated. (Work for a wider stride as you gain flexibility.) Gently lean forward and feel your body weight stretch your lower back and the insides and backs of your legs. Relax, lean back, and repeat. Now repeat the stretch over each leg.

Wide stride stretches

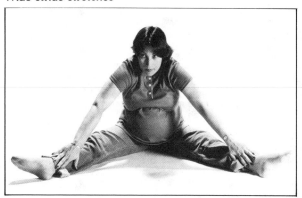 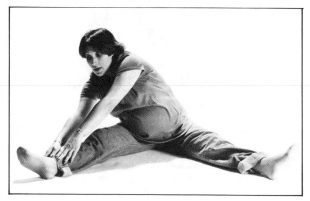

This exercise increases the strength and tone of your lower abdominal muscles, increases the flexibility of your back, promotes good pelvic alignment, relieves pelvic congestion, and helps prevent and relieve lower backache. There are four variations:

The pelvic tilt

1. Kneeling on all fours: With your hands directly under your shoulders and your knees directly under your hips, use your abdominal muscles to tuck your buttocks under and to round your lower back. Then slowly release your abdomen and allow your lower back to relax to a comfortable, almost flat position. Alternate these movements slowly with firm control.

The pelvic tilt

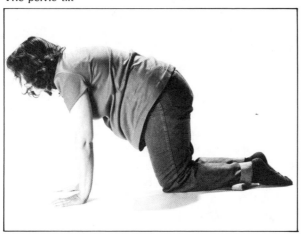 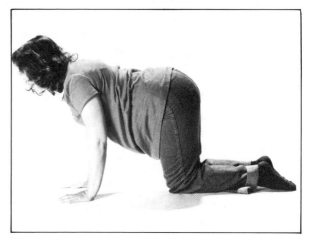

2. Lying on back: Bend your knees and place your feet flat on the floor. Inhale as you tighten your abdominal muscles, and tilt your pelvis up so that your lower back presses against the floor and your buttocks lift slightly. Do not push with your legs. Release your abdomen and inhale, allowing your pelvis to return slowly to a relaxed position. Alternate these movements with firm control.

3. Standing: With your feet slightly apart, place one hand under your abdomen and the palm of your other hand on the small of your back. Tighten your abdominal muscles firmly as you tuck your buttocks under, and tilt your pelvis up so that the curve in your back flattens out. Slowly release. Alternate these movements slowly with firm control.

4. Sitting: Sit on a hard chair and repeat the motions for the standing pelvic tilt.

New ways of moving

Another physical change that occurs during pregnancy is the release of the hormone relaxin which softens tissues, loosens joints, and affects the way you move. Here are some suggestions that can help you prevent fatigue, backache, tension, stress, falls, and injuries as you move through your days during pregnancy.

Walking and standing

You will be most comfortable walking tall with your shoulders back, chest out, and abdomen and buttocks tucked in. To have the feeling of walking tall, it may help to imagine yourself as a puppet. The puppeteer holds the strings from your head so your back is so straight that your feet barely touch the floor. When you must stand for long periods, put one foot on a stool or low shelf in order to maintain pelvic tilt. Putting one foot in front of the other and rocking from heel to toe will also help maintain pelvic tilt.

Sitting

To lower yourself into a chair, stand with one foot ahead of the other in front of the chair, your back leg touching the chair for balance. Place your hands on the edge of the chair for support and, using your leg muscles, lower yourself into the chair. Sit with a small stool under your feet to raise your knees slightly above hip level, and/or place a small pillow behind your hips below waist level to relieve back strain and fatigue. To rise from a chair, put your hands at your sides on the seat of the chair, and using your arm muscles rather than your back muscles, slide your bottom to the chair's edge. With one leg in front of the other, push off with your hands and arms and use your leg muscles to rise.

Bending and lifting

When you need to work at floor level or lift an object from the floor, squatting permits you to use your leg muscles to avoid straining your back muscles. Standing close to the object, put one foot slightly in front of the other and lower yourself slowly, keeping your pelvis tilted and your back straight. Pick up the object, hold it close to your body, and keeping your back straight, use your thigh muscles to rise. If this is difficult, drop to one knee and help yourself rise by pushing off against your other knee with one hand. Hold the object close to your body with the other arm.

Climbing stairs

To maintain your balance and to see the steps clearly during pregnancy, approach the stairs with your body turned at a slight angle to the steps. Keep your back straight, bend your knees slightly, and use a handrail for balance whenever possible. Going up, put your front foot firmly and completely on the step, push off with the toes of your back foot, and lift with your leg muscles. Coming down, put your whole foot on each step and use your thigh muscles for balance and control. Do not lean forward.

To rise from a lying position, bend your knees, roll to one side, and using your arms, push up to a sitting position. Swing your legs over the edge of the bed, and stand as though rising from a chair. If you are rising from the floor, bend your knees, roll to one side, and using your arms, push up to a sitting position. Next rotate to a kneeling position, then to kneeling on one knee and squatting on the other foot, and finally to a full squatting position. With one foot slightly in front of the other, rise using your thigh muscles and keeping your back straight.

Rising from a lying position

Rising from a lying position

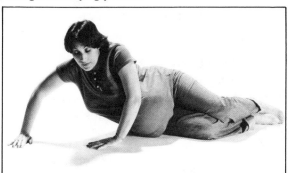 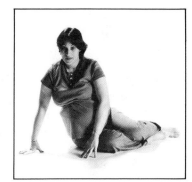 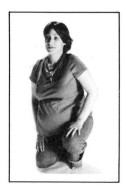

Physical discomforts

Although a woman's body is constituted to accommodate to the changes that occur during pregnancy, there are, nonetheless, a number of discomforts pregnant women experience. Below are some of the common discomforts of pregnancy and strategies for dealing with them.

There may be a tightening and relaxing of the uterine muscles prior to true labor. As your delivery date nears, these contractions may increase in frequency and strength. Using a focal point (focusing on a specific spot), massaging the abdomen, and taking a relaxing breath at the beginning and end of the contractions usually provide relief.

Braxton-Hicks contractions

Constipation Hard, though not necessarily infrequent, bowel movements may be another discomfort. The best ways to relieve and prevent constipation are to (1) increase the amount of roughage in your diet by eating lots of fruits, vegetables, and cereals; (2) drink three quarts of fluids daily; (3) exercise; and (4) eat prunes raw, stewed, or as juice. Sitting with your feet on a stool during bowel movements may help by giving your body better alignment. Do not use laxatives such as castor oil or epsom salts during pregnancy. Consult your health care provider for medication if constipation persists.

Fatigue In early and late pregnancy fatigue may occur. Be sure to get plenty of sleep at night and take extra naps during the day or after work if necessary.

Frequent urination You may need to urinate with increased frequency during early pregnancy and again during late pregnancy, when the baby's head moves down closer to your bladder. To relieve your bladder, urinate every two hours when you are awake. If pain, burning, or unusual frequency occur, consult your health care provider.

Groin pains You may feel mild, aching feelings or sharp, shooting pains on the sides of the lower abdomen. They occur intermittently throughout pregnancy and are probably caused by strain on the ligaments that support the uterus. Abdominal massage and rest may help.

Heartburn A common complaint in later pregnancy is heartburn. It is usually caused by regurgitation of acidic gastric juices into the esophagus, due to pressure from the enlarging uterus and sluggishness of the stomach. This causes a sharp, burning pain in the chest near the heart but does not involve the heart itself. It is aggravated by some types of foods such as coffee or fried foods. Drinking large amounts of water, eating several small meals a day, and eliminating aggravating foods may provide relief. Lying down at night, especially after eating, can make heartburn worse. Try elevating the head of your bed. You can use antacid preparations, but ask your health care provider for recommendations, since some preparations contain ingredients that should not be taken during pregnancy.

Sometimes called piles, hemorrhoids are varicose veins of the rectum. Especially common in late pregnancy, these purplish swellings around the anal opening or inside the rectum cause pain or bleeding during elimination. Since hemorrhoids are aggravated by constipation and diarrhea, try to avoid these two conditions by exercising and including plenty of roughage and fluids in your diet. The simplest comfort measure is sitting in a warm tub or sitz bath. You can also slowly tighten and slowly release the sphincter muscles around the anus. (See Kegel exercises in Chapter 5.) Any medication for hemorrhoids should be prescribed by your health care provider.

Hemorrhoids

Difficulty sleeping may be more pronounced in the last trimester of pregnancy. If sleeping on your stomach is the most comfortable position for you, go ahead and sleep on your stomach. It will not injure your baby. Consciously relaxing your muscles (see Chapter 5 for specific techniques) and taking a warm bath may help.

Insomnia

Slowed circulation or a calcium imbalance can cause leg cramps during pregnancy. You can relieve leg cramps by straightening your leg and flexing your foot without pointing your toes. If leg cramps are frequent or severe, consult your health care provider.

Leg cramps

During pregnancy, extra weight, postural changes, and the relaxation of joints and ligaments may cause lower-back pain. Because excessive strain or fatigue can aggravate lower-back pain, rest is one treatment that usually provides relief. Other comfort measures to try are (1) heating pads or warm baths; (2) moderate exercise to strengthen back muscles (see Posture check, Pelvic tilt, and Back stretching in this chapter); (3) wearing low-heeled shoes; (4) putting a bed board under your mattress; and (5) sleeping in a position other than on your stomach.

Minor lower-back pain

Symptoms of nausea usually ocur in early pregnancy and end by the fourth month. They are probably caused by hormonal changes. Although referred to as "morning" sickness, nausea and transient periods of vomiting can occur at any time of day. Eating small meals during the day or including a high protein snack at bedtime may help. Eating a cracker before getting out of bed sometimes relieves the problem of nausea in the morning.

Morning sickness

Shortness of breath In the latter months of pregnancy it is very common to experience shortness of breath, especially during exertion like stair climbing. Move slowly, avoid exertion, and walk tall with your chest out and abdomen and buttocks tucked in, since shortness of breath is caused by increased pressure on your diaphragm. (See Posture check in this chapter.)

Varicose veins A pregnant woman may notice veins that swell or dilate just under the skin, usually due to the increased pressure of weight gain. Preventive measures include leg elevation and sitting without crossing your legs. If varicose veins do occur, tell your health care provider, avoid standing for long periods of time, and rest frequently with your feet up. Support hose are also helpful, but remember to put them on before rising in the morning. Although varicose veins occur most often in the legs, they may also occur in the vulva (external genital organs).

Other changes Changes, not necessarily involving physical discomfort, that a pregnant woman may experience include (1) pigmentation changes around the nipples, on the face, and on the abdomen, including a dark, vertical line from the navel to the pubic bone (linea nigra); (2) striae, or stretch marks, on the abdomen, breasts, and thighs; and (3) increased breast size as the mammary glands prepare to produce milk. Breasts may also discharge colostrum, a watery, yellowish precursor of breast milk.

Warning signals and complications they may indicate

Almost every expectant mother experiences at least some of the discomforts of pregnancy. These discomforts are related to normal biological changes and are not particularly serious. There are other symptoms, however, that do indicate potentially serious conditions and these you should report immediately to your health care provider, who may call for one or more of the tests described in Chapter 2. Warning signals are

- Vaginal bleeding
- Persistent, severe vomiting
- Frequent urination, burning sensation with urination, or marked decrease in urine output

- Fever or chills
- Severe, continuous headache
- Visual disturbances
- Sudden weight gain (greater than five pounds in one week)
- Swelling or puffiness in the face or hands
- Steady abdominal pain or painful, persistent cramping
- Escape of fluid from the vagina (may be slow or sudden)
- Loss of or significant decrease in the baby's activity
- Sores in or near the genital area

When you report one of these warning signals to your health care provider, one of the following complications might be present.

Although not common, abruptio placenta occurs if the placenta or part of the placenta begins to separate from the wall of the uterus before the baby is born. This results in bleeding and/or very sudden, painful cramping. If significant maternal blood loss with subsequent loss of oxygen to the baby occurs, cesarean delivery usually becomes necessary. | *Abruptio placenta*

Another complication involves persistent, severe vomiting. Although many women experience some degree of nausea or vomiting during their pregnancy, it is uncommon for it to continue until they lose weight. Treatment for this condition usually includes administration of intravenous fluids to combat dehydration; intravenous glucose; possibly a fluid diet of high-caloric, high-vitamin substances through a nasal tube; and psychological support. | *Hyperemesis gravidarum*

Babies vary in degree of activity before birth just as they do afterwards, but women feel even the most inactive babies at least once a day. If more than one day goes by without feeling your baby move, notify your health care provider. | *Loss of fetal movement*

Although not common, a complication exists if the placenta partially or completely covers the cervix, which is the opening at the lower end of the uterus. Usually detected as the third trimester progresses and the cervix begins to thin and dilate, this condition may result in maternal bleeding and some loss of oxygen to the baby. After assessing the situation, perhaps through use of ultrasound, a health care provider may delay any action until the woman begins labor or reaches term. Sometimes the | *Placenta previa* placenta will remedy itself by growing or moving up the uterine wall. If the situation persists, however, a cesarean delivery is likely.

Premature rupture of the amniotic sac

A sudden escape of clear fluid from the vagina frequently indicates that the membranes, or bag of waters, have ruptured. Sometimes rupture occurs in an unmistakable gush, sometimes as a continuous, uncontrollable dribble. If you suspect that your membranes have ruptured, note whether or not the fluid is clear, whether or not the fluid has a disagreeable odor, and the time you first noticed the fluid. Call your health care provider immediately and relay this information. If you are unsure whether or not you are leaking amniotic fluid, a simple test may be performed at your health care provider's office or at the hospital. This determination is necessary, because without the protection of the amniotic sac and fluid, the baby is in danger of exposure to infection. Most health care providers prefer to deliver babies within 24 hours after the rupture of the membranes.

Toxemia

The condition called toxemia is characterized by some or all of the following symptoms: high blood pressure, protein in the urine, sudden weight gain, total body edema (swelling), headache, dizziness, and blurred vision. Usually, screening for toxemia during pregnancy occurs at each prenatal office visit by means of a blood-pressure check and sometimes a urine check. Treatment may begin with dietary changes and complete bed rest. If these measures do not reduce the problem, the health care provider may recommend hospitalization and, occasionally, early birth of the baby, which may occur by vaginal or cesarean delivery, depending on a number of circumstances.

There are other conditions that can occur, with few if any symptoms, during pregnancy. These potentially serious conditions include herpes simplex, blood incompatibility, and gestational diabetes.

Herpes simplex

Herpes is a viral illness that can become a long-term condition with flare-ups and remissions. It is first apparent when sores appear in or near a woman's genital area. When sores are present, the disease is contagious. If a vaginal birth occurs at this time, the baby is likely to contract the illness, and a large percentage of such babies can die. Therefore, a cesarean birth is usually crucial, followed by isolation of the baby after birth and limited contact between the baby and others in the nursery and post-partum unit. Some health care providers are equally cautious when the mother has a cold-sore lesion on her mouth, since this lesion is also caused by the herpes virus. Questions about herpes are routinely asked of all women checking into a hospital or birthing center for labor and delivery.

A woman with Rh negative blood who carries a baby with Rh positive blood can develop antibodies against the positive antigens in the baby's blood. This incompatibility develops at the time of birth when the baby's blood from the placenta mixes with the mother's blood. Giving the drug RhoGAM to the mother within 72 hours after delivery usually prevents the mother's blood from producing these antibodies. Some health care providers give women RhoGAM periodically throughout pregnancy on the slim chance that the mother's antibodies may develop and attack the baby's blood in utero. ABO incompatibility occurs occasionally when a mother with one major blood type (O+) gives birth to a baby with a different major blood type (A+), causing the mother to develop antibodies against the baby's blood. Babies with either ABO or Rh incompatibility experience jaundice, or hemolytic disease of the newborn (HDN). Babies with ABO-incompatible blood frequently have a more mild course of illness than babies with Rh incompatibility. Depending upon severity, both illnesses may be treated with phototherapy or blood-exchange transfusions.

Blood incompatibility

Since a woman's glucose tolerance is altered during pregnancy, some women develop high blood-sugar, or gestational diabetes. Some health care providers screen women for high blood-sugar during the last trimester, usually at 28 weeks, or earlier if there is a family history of diabetes. Women whose tests indicate abnormal glucose tolerance meet with a dietitian to set up a "modified diabetic diet" for the duration of the pregnancy. Glucose tolerance usually returns to normal after delivery. Some babies born to diabetic mothers may weigh nine pounds or more at birth. Such a baby may be too large to be delivered vaginally, necessitating a cesarean delivery.

Gestational diabetes

Emotional changes during pregnancy

Along with the joys and excitement of being pregnant you may also experience doubts, apprehensions, and a wide variety of other emotions. There is, after all, a certain amount of stress associated with pregnancy.

Hormones usually get all the blame for this stress. The body's hormonal levels are constantly changing throughout pregnancy, and consequent emotional changes vary greatly from woman to woman. The only definite finding from studies of the emotional effect of hormonal changes during pregnancy is that hormones do influence emotions.

Other physiological factors adding to stress during pregnancy are the increased size and weight of your uterus and baby, your increased blood volume, added demands on your heart and lungs, your enlarged abdomen, heavier breasts, stretch marks, and facial pigmentation changes. These changes make you look different and feel different about yourself. You may alternately feel glad, annoyed, disturbed, or anxious. These feelings may be reflected in dreams, mood swings, or nagging worries, but they should not cause despair. Conflicting emotions are normal, and dealing patiently with them helps prepare you for your new role as a parent. You may find it helpful to discuss your feelings with your spouse or mate, who is probably going through some emotional changes of his own.

The transition from lover/husband to lover/husband/father can be disturbing and frightening as well as exciting and challenging. Becoming a father can mean loss of freedom, added responsibility, a less active social life, and a changed relationship with you. (Two's company. Three's a crowd. Will he end up being the third party?) Ambivalent feelings about becoming fathers are common, but men are rarely encouraged to talk about them. Our society makes room for a pregnant woman's doubts about mothering but assumes that a man is automatically prepared to fulfill his role as father without question. When a couple is expecting a baby, people focus their attention on the mother. It seldom occurs to them to ask the father how he is feeling. Consequently, he may often feel somewhat resentful and left out. Fortunately, more men are refusing to be left out. They are attending childbirth classes and prenatal checkups, discussing their feelings, and taking a more active role in the birth process.

Sometimes when a man does not allow himself to express his concerns about his impending fatherhood even to himself, he experiences physical symptoms that parallel the discomforts of pregnancy: nausea, vomiting, weight gain, heartburn, back pain, and distended abdomen. W.H. Trethowan, a British psychiatrist, described and named this syndrome after a primitive ritual called the couvade. When a woman began labor, her husband would pretend to go through an exaggerated labor himself. He would groan, cry out in agony, and generally make as much commotion as he could, with the intent of drawing all the evil spirits away from his wife and child. Although our society does not formally subscribe to this ritual, the syndrome is very real. Research shows that about half of all expectant fathers show some symptoms.

Whenever we share feelings with another person, there is always the possibility of either decreasing or increasing tension and misunderstanding. In spite of the risks, it is essential that a couple expecting a baby communicate their most personal feelings with each other if they wish to grow together and maintain the kind of relationship that draws a family together.

Sexual changes during pregnancy

Many couples experience a new freedom from the concerns of contraception, once pregnancy is confirmed. Consequently, a couple's sexual relationship becomes more spontaneous and enjoyable. Sometimes, however, a woman's fatigue and nausea prevent her from feeling well enough to enjoy intercourse. If this is the case, physical closeness becomes especially important, along with the understanding that her fatigue and nausea will not last forever.

First trimester

Different studies come to differing conclusions regarding a woman's sexual desires and activities during the second trimester of pregnancy. Some studies show the second trimester to be the most sexually active period of pregnancy, because of a woman's decreased nausea, her acceptance of her pregnancy, her physical changes that mimic sexual arousal, and the leveling of her emotions. However, other studies show that, as pregnancy progresses, sexual activity decreases.

Second trimester

Having sexual intercourse at this point may become more of a challenge because of the woman's ever-expanding abdomen. Some couples experiment with and find new positions that are more comfortable. Others choose to express their love and affection through caressing and holding, resuming intercourse after the baby is born.

Third trimester

Since sexual expression is a vital element of a couple's relationship, a couple needs to talk together about their levels of desire, work hard together to maintain their relationship, and help each other grow both as people and as parents.

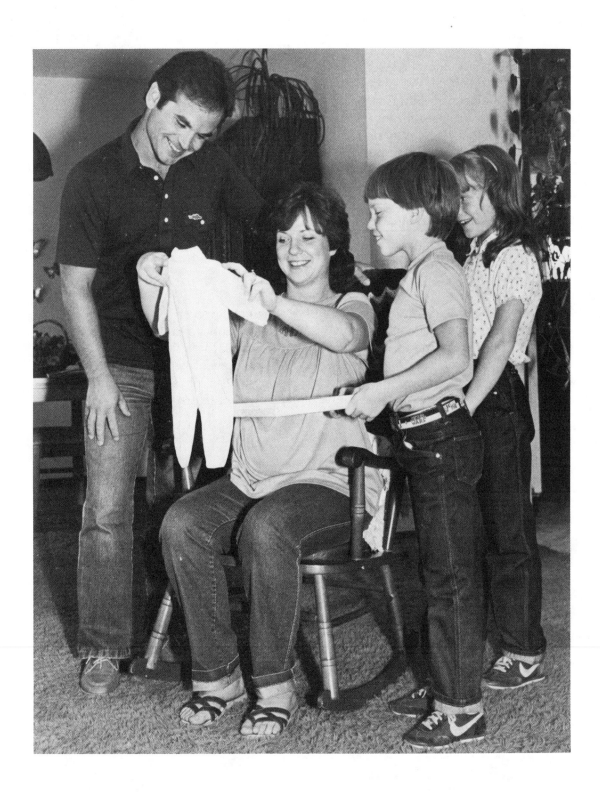

CHAPTER 4

Planning Ahead for Your Baby

Selecting a health care provider for your baby

If you do not already have a pediatrician—a physician specializing in the care of infants, children, and teenagers—you will want to select one to provide health care for your new baby. Along with treating your baby's illnesses, a pediatrician will help you understand and promote your baby's healthy growth and development. This process begins on your baby's first day of life in the hospital or birthing center when the pediatrician does a complete physical exam and shares the results with you.

Most visits to the pediatrician during your baby's first year will be "well" visits. The pediatrician will monitor your baby's health, growth, and development, alert you to subsequent phases of development, and administer preventive measures including immunizations. The pediatrician will also serve as a link between you and the medical community by making referrals to and clarifying information from specialists, and by admitting your child, writing orders, and interpreting hospital procedures if your child is hospitalized.

Selecting a pediatrician   Many parents interview and select a pediatrician during the last trimester of pregnancy. Most pediatricians welcome the opportunity to meet with parents before the baby's birth, but some charge for this preliminary visit. As you select a pediatrician, here are some issues you might consider:

- What are the pediatrician's qualifications—Board certification by the American Academy of Pediatrics or Board eligibility? (Board status indicates completion of specialized studies in pediatrics. It does not indicate competence.)

- Is the pediatrician affiliated with hospitals to which you would send your child for care? If your baby is born at a hospital with which the pediatrician is not affiliated, you will need to arrange care for your baby with another doctor until your baby is discharged.

- Does the pediatrician have a solo or group practice? In a solo practice, whom do you call nights, weekends, and holidays? In a group practice, what special services are offered? Does the practice include a pediatric nurse practitioner?

- How does the pediatrician feel about breast feeding? Bottle feeding? (If you are planning to breast feed, you may need a pediatrician's support if you encounter problems.)

- How soon will the pediatrician discharge your newborn baby from the hospital?

- What is the pediatrician's approach to infant feeding schedules? To demand feeding? To fixed routine feeding?

- What is the pediatrician's approach to prescribing medication? What role do parents have in deciding treatment?

- Will the pediatrician visit you and your newborn baby in the hospital?

- What kind of access will you have to the pediatrician—telephone consultation, house calls, answering service, or regular office hours?

- What fees does the pediatrician charge for office visits, immunizations, well-baby checkups, attendance at a cesarean birth, in-hospital visits?

- Is the atmosphere of the pediatrician's office crowded? Noisy? Quiet? Are there books and games for waiting children?

Upon making your selection, notify the pediatrician of your desire for services and your expected due date. Find out how the pediatrician wants to be notified of your baby's birth. The hospital nursery may take care of notification, but it is important to verify the policy with your pediatrician.

A pediatric nurse practitioner (PNP) is a registered nurse who has completed a program of study of the ambulatory health care of children from birth to adolescence. A PNP works in collaboration with a pediatrician and other members of the health care team to assess a child's physical, emotional, and social health and to provide treatment, counseling, and referral.

A pediatric nurse practitioner has both a hospital and pediatric office role. In the hospital, a PNP makes daily progress exams, evaluates the status of newborns and hospitalized children, follows up with pediatricians, and works extensively with parents. In the office, a PNP sees babies and children of all ages for routine well-child visits including physical exams, growth and development assessments, immunizations, counseling, and guidance. While the pediatrician diagnoses illness, the PNP and pediatrician collaborate on the follow-up care. A PNP is also available for telephone calls concerning well-child care problems including feeding, toilet training, and discipline.

A pediatric nurse practitioner

Some public health departments offer immunizations and well-baby exams at greatly reduced rates or at no cost. Plan ahead by calling your local health department to find out the services they provide, when services are scheduled, and any restrictions that apply, such as age requirements.

Health care services at reduced cost

Feeding your baby

Providing nourishment for your baby will be one of your new responsibilities. There are two basic choices you can make—breast feeding or bottle feeding. Nutrition may be a major consideration when you decide which feeding method to use. Some experts believe that there is no conclusive evidence proving either method nutritionally superior. Other experts, however, emphatically state that breast milk is superior to any formula. To decide which choice will be best for you, you will want to consider the relative merits of each method. These merits are summarized as follows:

A case for breast feeding

Convenient	Requires no preparation. Requires no special equipment or storage (unless milk is expressed into a bottle by mother for future use).
Healthy	Provides antibodies that partially protect baby from infection for the first six months or longer.

Child-centered	Allows babies to control amount they drink.
Nutritious	Provides a complete nutritional package—raw, fresh, and sterilized. Each mother's milk is biochemically unique to suit the needs of her baby. Content of mother's milk adapts to the baby's growing needs.
Digestible	Provides milk that digests easily and rapidly and therefore prevents some feeding problems, allergic reactions, and constipation.
Economical	Is less costly than bottle feeding.
Nurturing	Can develop a unique bond between mother and baby when they share the satisfaction and physical intimacy of breast feeding.

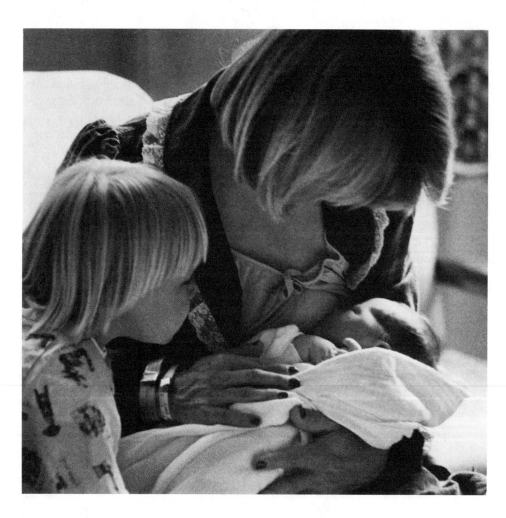

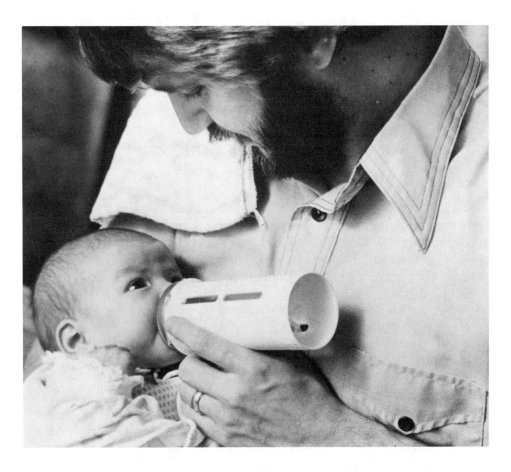

A case for bottle feeding

Comfortable   Can be done without exposing the breasts. Mothers do not experience discomfort of enlarged, tender, leaking breasts.

Convenient   Can be done anywhere by anyone. Fathers, siblings, relatives, babysitters, friends, can help with feedings, freeing the mother from total responsibility for the baby's nourishment.

Accurate   Accurately indicates the amount of formula a baby drinks. This is reassuring to many parents who are anxious about whether their baby is getting enough nourishment.

If you are undecided about which feeding method is best for you, discuss both methods with knowledgeable individuals, read some books about feeding (see Suggested Reading), or contact the local chapter of La Leche League International, an organization devoted to the support of mothers who breast feed. Selecting the feeding method that feels most comfortable to you will help convey your confidence and contentment to your newborn baby.

Deciding about eye protection and circumcision

Eye protection In the United States, the public health law requires babies to receive protective drops in their eyes shortly after birth. These drops effectively kill venereal-disease-causing bacteria that may have come in contact with the baby's eyes as the baby passed through the birth canal. Without treatment the baby could become blind. Even though most pregnant women do not have venereal disease, each state has laws calling for medication to prevent infectious eye disease in newborn babies. These laws apply also to babies born by cesarean delivery, since infection can spread to the baby's eyes merely through the early rupture of the amniotic sac.

In recent years parents have expressed concern about the negative effects of silver nitrate treatment—a burning sensation in the baby's eyes, swollen eyelids, and the blurring of the baby's vision which may interfere with the bonding process. (In some cases, silver nitrate is administered at the latest time legally possible after birth. This allows time for parents to interact with their newborn baby immediately after delivery.)

Alternatives to silver nitrate treatment are available, but you may need to ask for them specifically. Tetracycline and erythromycin ointments, for example, are as effective against venereal disease as silver nitrate is and do not burn or cause the same type of pain that silver nitrate apparently does.

Since there are no effective tests to prove the existence of eye infection in babies before delivery, and since available post-delivery laboratory tests require 48 hours to produce results, hospitals must regard all mothers as potential eye-infection carriers and, therefore, must protect all infants against possible eye infection.

You may want to discuss this information with your health care provider during one of your prenatal visits. You will then need to mention your preference for silver nitrate, tetracycline, or erythromycin to the nurse in the labor-delivery area when you are admitted to the hospital or birthing center for labor and delivery.

Another common procedure for a newborn baby boy is the surgical removal of the foreskin that covers the tip of the penis. If parents decide to have their son circumcised, the procedure is usually performed by the obstetrician or pediatrician within the first few days after birth.

Historically, circumcision has been done for religious and cultural reasons. Until recently, there seemed to be several medical indications for circumcision at birth, including the prevention of cancer of the penis. However, this extremely rare type of cancer, along with infection under the foreskin, can be prevented in uncircumcised males by proper hygiene. There is also no indication that uncircumcised men promote cancer of the cervix or vagina in their sexual partners. The inability to retract the foreskin, phimosis, is a condition that may occur in uncircumcised, adult males who have poor personal hygiene.

According to the American Academy of Pediatrics, "there are no medical indications for routine circumcision. A program of education leading to continuing good personal hygiene would offer all the advantages of routine circumcision without the attendant surgical risk. Therefore, circumcision of the male newborn cannot be considered an essential component of adequate total health care."

As you think about circumcision, you may want to consider whether or not other males in the family are circumcised. Some psychologists believe that an adolescent boy feels more comfortable when his penis looks like those of his peers. There are several disadvantages to circumcision, including the pain of the operative procedure, the risk of infection and excessive bleeding, and the baby's increased irritability right after the operation. You will want to consider before delivery the advantages and disadvantages of circumcision. Talk with your health care provider and pediatrician so that you can be confident of making an informed decision.

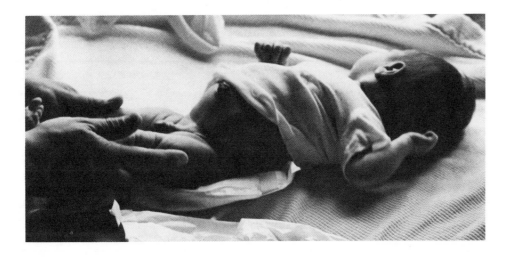

Outfitting your baby: Equipment and clothing

The following lists will help you think about the equipment and clothing you want to gather for your baby before you go to the hospital.

Equipment

Car safety seat*

Crib (regular, portable, bassinet, or cradle)

Changing table (or vinyl pad on top of small chest of drawers)

Reclining infant seat (Some car seats can double as a play or feeding seat.)

Cold-steam vaporizer (Safer than hot-steam, it humidifies the air during winter making it easier for baby to breathe if congested.)

Stroller (A carriage is a nice luxury.)

Baby carrier (front and/or back)

Diaper bag (A beach bag or large purse works well.)

Diaper pail (Diaper services provide a pail during service.)

Night light

Bottle feeding equipment (several 8-ounce bottles, 4-ounce bottles, nipples, caps, disposable bags, if necessary)

Brush and comb

Baby rectal thermometer (The hospital may give you one.)

Layette

4-6 undershirts

4-6 gowns, kimonos, or sack sets

4-6 pairs waterproof pants (if using cloth diapers)

---

*Before you enter the hospital, borrow, rent, or purchase a car safety seat so your baby's first ride will be a safe one. Correct, consistent use of a safety seat is the only way to protect your baby against the number one threat to your baby's life—car crashes.

The best safety seat is one that meets current federal safety standards and one that you are willing to use properly every time your baby rides in a motor vehicle. If you are purchasing or borrowing a previously owned seat, be sure that it meets current federal safety standards and that all the parts are intact.

For assistance in selecting and using your baby's car safety seat, contact the local Child Passenger Safety Association, County Health Department, or State Highway Safety Program.

4-6 stretch suits (depending on season)

6-7 dozen cloth diapers for home washing

6 diaper pins

1 box cotton balls or cotton-tipped applicators

1 tube cream, ointment, or petroleum jelly

1-2 baby washcloths and towels

1 waterproof mattress cover (if mattress isn't waterproof)

1-2 mattress pads

3 crib sheets

4-6 waterproof pads (puddle pads for air-drying baby's bottom, to put on changing table)

1 set of crib bumper pads

2 buntings or blanket sleepers (depending on season)

1 thermal blanket

4-6 receiving blankets

Preparing for your hospital stay

Having a baby, like any other major change in household routine, benefits from advance planning. Here are some strategies to help you feel that things are still under control:

- Plan for upcoming holidays by purchasing gifts or cards before you go to the hospital.

- Purchase birth announcements appropriate for either sex, address and stamp them.

- Fix casseroles and other dishes that can be frozen. Stock the kitchen with ingredients for easily prepared meals.

- Make arrangements for care of older children during your absence.

- If necessary, arrange for household help for when you return from the hospital. This person can concentrate on the household chores, leaving you free to care for your baby, and could be the father, a relative, a close friend, or a neighborhood teenager.

- If you wish, arrange with the local health department for a visit by a public health nurse who will examine your baby and discuss any concerns.
- Tour the maternity area of the hospital where you will deliver.
- Become familiar with the route and the amount of time it takes to get to the hospital.
- If you plan to have rooming-in, learn about the hospital's rooming-in policies.
- Set out clothes you want to wear home from the hospital. Because your abdomen will still be somewhat enlarged, plan to wear a loose-fitting or maternity outfit.
- Set out clothes for your baby to wear home from the hospital.
- Buy a large box of sanitary pads which you will need for a while during your recovery at home.
- To avoid last minute rushing, pack your suitcase several weeks before your due date.

Things to pack for the hospital

Large suitcase

(Leave this one in the car. Have your labor partner bring it later to your postpartum room.)

Nightgowns—2 (open fronts for nursing mothers)

Bras—2 or 3 (nursing bras if you plan to breast feed)

Bathrobe

Slippers

Toilet articles

Your own pillow if you prefer it (in a colorful case so it does not get lost)

Sanitary pads and belt (most hospitals provide them)

Small suitcase or goody bag

(Take this into the labor room.)

Warm socks—1 pair

Lollipops—2 or 3

Lip balm

Pencil and paper

Eyeglasses (if worn)

Tennis balls for backrubs

Watch with a second hand

Picture or object to use as focal point

Shower cap (if the labor room has a shower)

Small paper sack to use in case of hyperventilation

Snack for labor partner

Change for the telephone

Cornstarch or unscented oil for light abdominal massage and backrubs

Preparing older children for a new family member

Regardless of their ages, children sense ahead of time that something unusual is going to happen in their family. Therefore, along with telling children about an anticipated baby, you can also prepare them for the changes that will occur. Some changes, like sleeping in a big bed while baby uses the crib, are easier for children to accept if you make the switch to the new bed well in advance of the baby's arrival. Other issues like your hospital or birthing center stay may make more sense to discuss with your children in the month preceding your expected delivery date. In addition to reassuring your older children that you will still love them and have time for them after the baby is born, here are some other strategies you might find helpful, depending on the ages and needs of your older children:

Before the baby comes

- Refer to baby as "our baby" rather than "the baby," "Mommy's baby," or "the new baby."

- Let older children prepare for baby's arrival by helping select baby's name, helping make the birth announcements, and helping choose baby's homecoming outift.

- Take children along on a prenatal health care visit to listen to baby's heartbeat and learn about labor and delivery and how babies develop before birth.

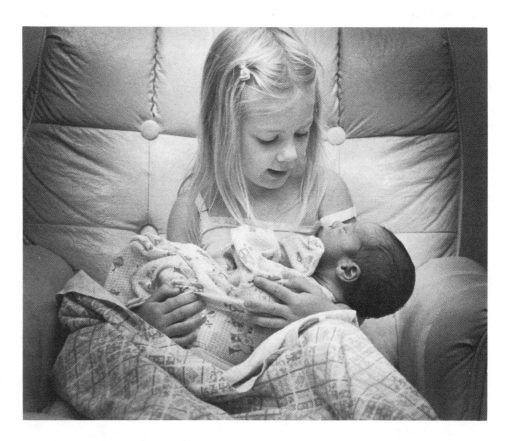

- If possible, visit a home with an infant, so that your children realize that their baby will not be an instant playmate.

- Talk with your children about the advantages of a baby of either sex and the unpredictability of a baby's sex.

- Show older children their own baby pictures. Explain what it was like when they were born, fed, diapered, and washed, and how, like them, baby will not smile or talk or have any hair or teeth.

- Make any major room changes or additions well before baby arrives. This is especially important if you are planning to move baby into a crib or room currently used by an older child.

- Before baby arrives, allow older children to play with baby's toys, handle baby's clothes, look in drawers, and explore the changing table. By the time baby comes, the newness of these baby items will have diminished and you will have avoided some of the over-stimulation that often accompanies baby's first days home.

- About four to six weeks ahead of time, make arrangements for older children's care while you are in the hospital. Discuss your plans with them. If possible, have them cared for at home by father, grandmother, grandfather, or a familiar babysitter. Otherwise, arrange care in another familiar home. A trial overnight stay before baby arrives may ease the situation.

- Write out a schedule of your children's usual activities and routines for the person caring for them while you are away.

- Prepare your children for the fact that you will be away while you are having baby. You may wish to prepare a special letter or tape recording or leave a picture of yourself for your children to keep.

- Encourage your children to help you pack your suitcase. Ask children to loan you a picture or toy you can keep in the hospital.

- Before baby arrives, teach your children independent, age-appropriate behavior (playing by themselves, toileting, dressing). It is unrealistic to expect independent behaviors to develop immediately and spontaneously once baby arrives.

- Buy your children dolls or stuffed animals they can care for just as mother and father care for baby.

- Using a doll or stuffed animal, teach your children how to hold a baby gently but securely.

- Purchase a few gifts for your children, so when visitors bring a gift for baby, older children have gifts too.

- Prepare for the first day home from the hospital. Decide who will be there, who will hold baby, who will be with older children. Making plans as specific as possible will minimize anxiety and help create a memorable homecoming.

- Enroll in the class "Becoming Brothers and Sisters."

During the birth process

A current trend in this country is toward having older children present during labor, during delivery, or shortly after birth. While some hospitals are flexible in trying to meet families' desires, others are not. If you wish to make special arrangements for your children to participate in the birth process, talk first with your health care provider who may or may not be comfortable with the idea. If your health care provider is willing, you will then need to make arrangements with the head nurse of the hospital's labor and delivery unit. If you are not satisfied with the options the head nurse offers, your only recourse may be to choose another hospital offering broader options.

If you are unsure about having your children present during birth, here are some issues to consider. How comfortable will your children be seeing you partially clothed? How old are your children? What are their interests, concerns, and responses to new situations? How much advance preparation are you willing to do so they will be less frightened? If you do decide to include your children in the birth process, be sure they understand that they may have to leave at any time due to unpredictable circumstances. Include a support person, other than your labor partner, whom the children can turn to for any reason during the birth process. Allow your children to select their own physical space during the event, have them bring activities that will help keep them occupied, and try to have someone take photographs to help you recall this unique family experience.

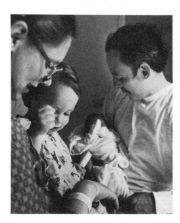 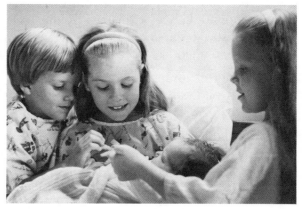

At the hospital after the birth   In the interest of providing family-centered birthing, many hospitals provide regularly scheduled times for children to visit mother and baby. Although this policy varies among hospitals, it frequently means that children can come to the mother's room as often as twice a day, as long as visiting children are free of colds, coughs, fevers, or recent exposure to childhood illnesses like chicken pox. Healthy children are asked to wash their hands, put on a hospital gown over their clothing, and visit only with you and baby.

Since separation from mother can be stressful, especially for children between the ages of one and four, hospital visits can help reduce your children's anxiety about where you really are and can assure your children that you still remember and love them. During these visits, it may help children to visit with you first and then go with you to the nursery.

At the end of the visit, a toddler or preschooler may protest loudly. Such protest is normal and healthy and nurses are accustomed to it. Once out of your sight, your toddler or preschooler will recover rapidly.

Here are some other strategies that might help your older children feel more comfortable about your hospital stay:

- Telephone your children daily while you are in the hospital. These calls will reassure you as well as the children.

- Have your older children give something special (candy, gum) to friends announcing the baby's birth.

- Save little packets of sugar and jelly from hospital food trays as souvenirs for your children to use at home.

- Tape a picture of your older children to baby's bassinet to help them recognize baby when they come to visit.

- Prepare a birthday cake or cupcakes and have a party when the older children visit in the hospital. Here is a chance to talk about what *birth*day means.

Once home from the hospital, one of the best things you can do for yourself and your family is to relax and allow everyone including yourself the time they need to adjust to family life with a new family member. Together, aided by time, a sense of humor, and an acceptance of each other's strengths and weaknesses, you will face new demands and new opportunities for growth and development. Here are some strategies that might be helpful to you and your family:

Home from the hospital: Reestablishing family life

- Allow older children to be helpful: fold diapers; refill baby's tray; help dress, burp, and feed baby; put lotion on baby's arms and legs.

- Encourage older children to smile and talk to baby, especially when baby is fussy. Acknowledge baby's positive response.

- Teach older children to hold baby. If you have a toddler or preschooler, begin by taking her or his hand and showing how and where to touch baby. By making a toddler's first approach to baby positive, you can avoid a strong "no."

- Encourage older children to share some but not all toys with baby. Provide space in your home that belongs solely to the older children.

- Avoid giving older children responsibilities concerning baby beyond their capabilities.

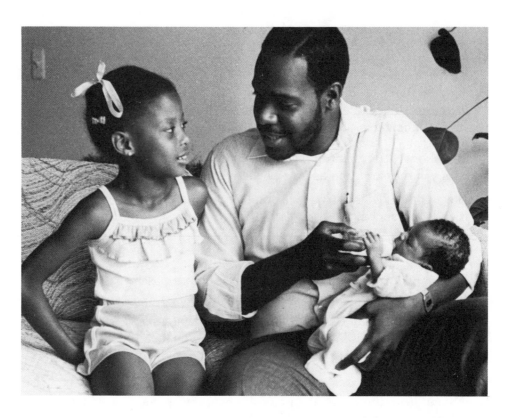

- Spend some time alone with each child every day to make older children more tolerant of the time you spend with baby.

- You may wish to postpone involving older children in new activities, independent of you, outside the home. Older children might interpret these activities as your desire to "get rid" of them. Once assured over time that you still want them, however, they will be ready to venture out again.

- Be flexible. Older children may balk at well-established routines (going to nursery school, for example) after baby arrives. This behavior is normal and will disappear in time.

- During feeding times encourage older children to snuggle close to you for a story or a special talk while you feed baby.

- If your preschooler asks to nurse, too, allow her or him to try, or express some milk into a cup. If you maintain a matter-of-fact approach, your child will too and will soon lose interest.

- Reminisce with older children about their own "babyhood." Express pride in their growth and development. Reinforce the advantages of growing up.

- Praise older children's positive behavior. Try to ignore their negative behavior. (Some children may temporarily regress to "being a baby.")

- Try to organize activities the whole family can enjoy together—walks, trips to the park, drives.

- Share care for baby and older children with father. Try to divide tasks so that both parents share in the joy (and the drudgery!) of each of the children. In this way, children can learn early in life that fathers take care of babies, too.

- Enroll in a parent discussion group. Share your experiences and gain support from other parents.

Regardless of all your preparations, there will be times when the older children feel left out and think you do not love them anymore. They may hit or be angry with the baby. When this occurs, here are some strategies to try:

- Get down on your child's eye level, hold the child's hands firmly, and say something like, "I know you are angry, but I will not allow you to hurt baby. If baby cried and was hurt because of you, you wouldn't feel good either. When you feel this way again tell me, so we can talk about it."

- Encourage your child to talk about negative feelings.

- It may be helpful to say, "Do you need me to hold you right now?" or "Do you need something from me?"

- You may need to isolate the child for a short time, using a timer, after explaining why the behavior is not allowed. After an isolation period, hold your child and give special attention.

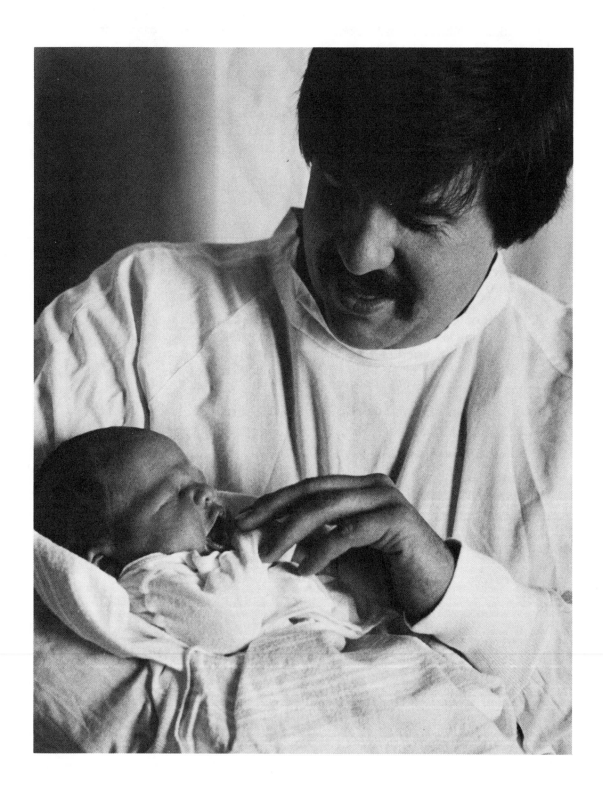

CHAPTER 5

Preparing for Labor and Delivery

Limbering exercises

Prenatal exercise keeps your body in good physical shape, maintains muscle tone, and hastens your recovery after childbirth. Because the uterus is an involuntary muscle, there are no exercises that will shorten labor. However, prenatal exercise helps you feel good during pregnancy, and being in good physical shape helps you relax during labor.

The following exercises are designed to condition your neck and shoulders, back, abdomen, pelvis, and legs. To prevent strain and fatigue, do these exercises slowly and start by doing each one five times a day unless otherwise indicated. Also, try to include these movements in your normal daily routine.

This exercise aids neck and shoulder relaxation during pregnancy and labor. To begin, sit on a firm surface with your back straight, your knees bent, and your ankles crossed or as nearly crossed as you can get them (in tailor position). (1) Roll your head gently forward toward your chest, over your right shoulder, back, over your left shoulder, and forward toward your chest again. After repeating this five times, repeat the sequence in the reverse direction five times. Breathe regularly. (2) Rotate your shoulders up, back, down, and forward. Repeat, and then do the sequence in the reverse direction. Again, remember to breathe regularly.

Head and shoulder circles

Arm and shoulder reaches For upper body and shoulder flexibility, sit in either a wide stride or tailor position and stretch in the following ways: (1) Reach over your head and stretch first one arm and then the other, as if you were trying to touch the ceiling. Inhale while relaxed, then exhale and stretch until you feel your whole side lengthen. To get more stretch, bend your torso toward the side opposite the arm you are reaching with. Reach toward the wall instead of the ceiling. (2) Start with your arms straight out at shoulder level. Inhale and press your arms backward, drawing your shoulder blades together. Exhale and "hug" yourself by crossing your arms in front of you, wrapping them as far around yourself as you can. Repeat five times.

Back stretching This exercise promotes lower-back muscle flexibility which is needed for correct posture. (See instructions in Chapter 3.)

Upper abdominal control This exercise strengthens the upper abdominal muscles used for pushing during the second stage of labor. (1) Lie on your back with your knees bent and your feet flat on the floor. Curl your head and shoulders off the floor as if you were trying to look over your abdomen. Feel the tension in your upper abdominal muscles. Lower your head and shoulders slowly to the floor. (2) Lie on your back and exhale through your mouth as if to blow out a candle. Continue to blow until you run out of air. You will feel your upper abdominal muscles tighten. Repeat.

Kegel exercise This exercise teaches you to relax the pelvic floor muscles, which help prevent involuntary urine leakage. It also strengthens the muscles that support the bladder, urethra, vagina, uterus, and rectum. To begin, slowly tighten the urethra as though to stop the flow of urine. Next, tighten the muscles that surround the vagina and feel your pelvic floor lift. Finally, tighten the sphincter muscle around the anus. Hold for five seconds, and slowly release. Repeat this exercise ten times, three times a day. Concentrate on the feelings of tension and release. This feeling of relaxed pelvic floor muscles is one you will want to maintain during delivery, as you push your baby out.

Perineal massage You or your partner can do this massage for five minutes a day beginning about six weeks before your due date. Lying in a semi-seated position against some pillows, begin by looking in a mirror at your perineum (tissues around the anus and vulva) so you know what you are doing. Dip your fingers into a clean vegetable oil or vitamin E oil and rub the oil into the perineum and lower vaginal wall. If you are doing the massage yourself, it is probably easiest to use your thumbs. Your partner can use the index fingers. Put your fingers three inches into the vagina and press downward toward the rectum. Maintaining steady pressure, slide your fingers upward along the sides of the vagina, moving them in a rhythmic U movement. This will stretch the vaginal tissue, the muscles surrounding the vagina, and the skin of the perineum. In the beginning your perineum will feel tight, but with time and practice the tissue will relax and stretch. As you become comfortable with this massage, use enough pressure until the perineum begins to sting. Later you will feel this sensation as the baby's head is born and your perineum stretches around it. If you have any questions after trying this massage, ask your health care provider.

The pelvic tilt

This exercise increases the strength and tone of your lower abdominal muscles, increases the flexibility of your back, promotes good pelvic alignment, relieves pelvic congestion, and helps prevent and relieve lower backache. (See instructions in Chapter 3.)

Thigh limbering

Sit on a firm surface with your back straight, your knees bent, and the soles of your feet together and as close to your body as possible. Put your hands on your ankles and inhale. Exhale as you use your leg muscles to lower your knees gently toward the floor. You should feel a strong pull on your inner thighs. Repeat.

Wide stride stretches

This exercise promotes leg and lower-back flexibility. (See instructions in Chapter 3.)

Leg elevation

This position helps prevent varicose veins and muscle cramps by improving blood circulation to the legs and pelvis. Lie on the floor, on your back, with your feet against the wall or with your legs on a chair, a cushion, a rolled blanket, or any other object that elevates your feet above the level of your heart. Put a folded towel or pillow under your hips. Rest in this position for five to ten minutes as often as you can. You may find this position especially beneficial before retiring.

Comfort measures to practice

The following comfort measures are techniques your labor partner can use to help make your labor as comfortable as possible. You may also find them helpful during pregnancy. Many women and their partners incorporate these comfort measures into their daily practice sessions where they serve two purposes: (1) to relax the mother and (2) to condition mother and partner to use comfort measures in addition to active relaxation and patterned breathing as responses to a contraction.

Back massage   Your partner can give back massages in a variety of ways on any part of your back, using mineral oil or talcum powder to decrease friction, if you wish. To release tension in your neck and shoulders, your partner can massage your upper back along your spine with the thumbs, or stroke your neck and shoulders firmly with the fingertips. Your partner can give a general back massage by stroking up and out from your spinal column with palms, fingertips, a paint roller, a wooden rolling pin covered with a hand towel, or a hollow rolling pin filled with ice water. Your partner can also do a figure-eight massage side to side over your buttocks, crossing at the sacrum, or up and down from the small of your back to your tailbone. Using the heel of the hand or side of the fist, your partner applies more pressure at the sacrum and less pressure over the buttocks and back.

Back pressure   Your partner can apply pressure to the area over your tailbone, using the palm of the hand. You can apply back pressure yourself by leaning on your fists or on a firm object like a tennis ball. You can also apply counter-pressure by sitting back to back with your partner.

Effleurage   This is a French term for the gentle, rhythmic, circular, fingertip stroking of the abdomen, back, or thighs. You or your partner can do the stroking.

The passive pelvic tilt   Your partner can use this technique when your back aches during labor. As you lie on your side on the edge of the bed, your partner approaches you from behind and stands behind your hips. Your partner's hand that is closer to your head goes on your hip for stabilization, fingertips pointing toward your toes. The partner's other hand goes on your sacrum (tailbone). Your partner leans forward on the outside leg (farther from the bed) applying pressure to your sacrum, then backward on the inside leg (closer to the bed) releasing pressure. As your partner's weight shifts

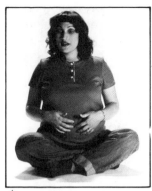
Effleurage

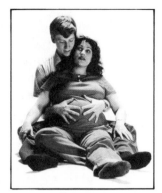
Partner effleurage

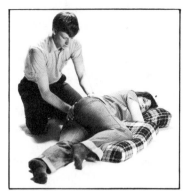
Passive pelvic tilt

slowly and rhythmically from leg to leg, your pelvis tilts. Your partner can also approach you from the front. As you lie on your side, your partner stands at your hips. Your partner puts the hand closer to your head on your hip. Your partner's other hand goes on your sacrum. Your partner then shifts from leg to leg, tilting your pelvis as described. If you are lying on your back, your partner stands beside you, facing your feet. Both of your partner's hands go under your buttocks. As your partner shifts forward and back from leg to leg, your pelvis tilts. Alternatively, your partner can loop a towel under your buttocks and tilt your pelvis by pulling up on the towel.

A compress (towel or cloth dipped in water and wrung out) is especially soothing during back labor. Your partner can apply a compress to your tailbone while using the passive pelvic tilt. Your partner can apply a warm compress over your pubic bone to relieve the sensation that your cervix is stretching. Alternating hot and cold compresses every 15-30 minutes can also provide comfort.

A cold or warm compress

Your partner can help you release tensed muscles by stroking your legs, arms, feet, and hands.

Stroking the extremities

Active relaxation exercises

Active relaxation exercises, also known as neuromuscular control exercises, are based on conditioned response and involve the following physiological sequence of events: the human brain receives a signal, interprets the sensation, and selects a response. During labor, a woman's uterus contracts, emitting a signal to the brain which interprets the signal and gives a response. In a woman unprepared for childbirth, this response is usually muscular tension. In a woman trained in the Lamaze method, the response is often active relaxation. Although relaxation is often associated with sleep and the loss of muscle activity, active relaxation involves being awake, being aware of sensations and external stimuli, and making conscious choices about how to respond.

A conditioned response is a learned or practiced reaction to a specific stimulus. By practicing the exercises described in this chapter, you can condition yourself to respond to a contraction by relaxing voluntary muscles, breathing in a specific pattern, and employing appropriate comfort measures. You will need to practice these exercises over and over again, however, until your response to a contraction becomes second nature.

Active breathing exercises condition your body to relax during labor and, thus, to labor more comfortably and efficiently. Active relaxation also enables your circulatory system to work more effectively at carrying oxygen to your uterus.

Scheduling practice sessions

(1) Practice for ten minutes a day at least five days a week. (2) Practice at least three times a week with your partner. (3) Practice when you have time and when you are not too tired.

Preparing for practice sessions

(1) Empty your bladder and bowel. (2) Wear loose clothing. If the room is cool, wear something warm, since cold air causes muscles to contract. You may want to remove glasses, jewelry, and gum, which can be distracting. (3) Lie down on a comfortable, firm surface with your joints slightly flexed. Use cushions where you need them for support—a pillow or a rolled towel underneath your lower back, pillows underneath your arms, and pillows underneath your knees and feet.

During the first weeks of practice, lie on your back on the floor. Place a small pillow or rolled towel under your right hip. This will tilt you slightly to your left, displacing the weight of your uterus from the deep blood vessels along your spine. It will also keep you from feeling nauseated or light-headed, make it easier for you to feel and release muscle tension, and allow your partner to see and check what you are doing.

In the later weeks of practice and during labor, you may find that a side-lying position is more comfortable. Use pillows underneath your head, knees, and uterus.

During practice sessions and at other times as well, you, the partner, will learn to recognize and release tension in the mother. Watch for tension in her eyes, mouth, shoulders, neck, and hands. Clues that indicate tension are sudden movement (however slight), hardening of the muscles, and rigidity in an extremity. Use comfort measures, particularly back massage, back pressure, and passive pelvic tilt as needed to help her relax and feel comfortable. Note the position she assumes while sleeping and remind her of it during practice, since it is probably a comfortable position for her. During practice sessions, you will give the directions indicated in the exercises, telling the mother which muscles to tense and relax. Be definite and consistent in your use of the terms "tense" or "contract" and "release" or "relax."

The partner's role in active relaxation

Relaxation causes your blood pressure to drop. Therefore, to prevent dizziness when you rise at the end of a relaxation session, stretch your arms over your head, roll over on your side, sit up slowly, and rise slowly to your feet.

Ending an exercise session

Do this exercise at the beginning of every relaxation session. Begin with a full, deep, relaxing breath. Inhale as deeply as you can through your nose, relax your lips, and release the air through your mouth as if you were sighing. Repeat. As you do this, concentrate on relaxing your entire body. Breathe deeply, slowly, and quietly, in and out through your nose. At all times concentrate on specific muscle areas and learn to recognize the specific sensations associated with relaxation versus tension.

Toe-to-head release

Exercise 1: Toe-to-head release

Direction	Action
Tense and release your feet.	Flex and tense your feet, wiggle your toes, and rotate your ankles. Release the muscles in your feet. Feel each foot become limp and relaxed.
Tense and release your legs.	Slowly stretch your legs by pushing with your heels (not your toes). Release your calves and thighs, taking the same amount of time it took to tense them. Feel relaxation spread to your hips and abdomen. Continue to breathe quietly through your nose.
Tense and release your trunk.	Tense your abdomen, buttocks, perineum, and chest, and slowly release them.

Tense and release your shoulders.	Press your shoulders into the surface you are lying on. Rotate your shoulders in a circle. Repeat three times and feel the release of tension.
Tense and release your arms.	Stretch your arms and lock your elbows. Release your elbows and feel relaxation spread from your upper arms to your lower arms.
Tense and release your hands.	Stretch your fingers and make a fist. Repeat three times and release. Feel relaxation spread from your hands to your fingers.
Tense and release your neck.	Tense your neck and gently roll your head in a circle. Repeat three times, then reverse direction. Feel relaxation in your neck.
Tense and release your face.	Tense your face, feeling tension spread from the jaw to the cheeks to the forehead. Slowly release your face and feel relaxation spread from your jaw to your tongue, cheeks, eyes, forehead, and scalp.
Keep your whole body released.	Listen to your heartbeat. Take a deep, relaxing breath. As you exhale, you will feel a sense of lightness and warmth. You have released deeply embedded muscle tension.

Individual muscle tension and relaxation   Assume a comfortable supported position. Focus on a specific spot or object. Take a relaxing breath. Concentrate on how your muscles feel as you tense and release them.

Exercise 2: Individual muscle tension and relaxation

Direction	**Action**
Tense and release your right hand.	Tense your right hand and slowly release it.
Tense and release your right forearm.	Tense your right forearm while the rest of your arm remains released. Slowly release your right forearm.

Tense and release your right upper arm.	Tense only your right upper arm. Slowly release it.
Tense and release your right shoulder.	Tense your right shoulder and slowly release it.
Tense and release your left hand, left forearm, left upper arm, left shoulder.	Tense and slowly release your left hand, forearm, upper arm, and shoulder, isolating each muscle group. Take a slow, relaxing breath.
Tense and release your left foot.	Tense your left foot and slowly release it.
Tense and release your left lower leg.	Tense only your left lower leg and slowly release it.
Tense and release your entire left leg.	Tense your entire left leg and slowly release it.
Tense and release your right foot, right lower leg, entire right leg.	Tense and slowly release the muscles of your right foot and leg.
Keep your body released.	Take a slow, relaxing breath. Take another slow, relaxing breath. Your body should be completely relaxed. Concentrate and think, "Total muscle release, body relaxation."
Your feet are completely relaxed.	Think about your feet being completely relaxed.
Your legs are completely relaxed.	Think about your legs being completely relaxed.
Your bottom is completely relaxed.	Think about your bottom being completely relaxed.
Your back is completely relaxed.	Think about your back being completely relaxed.
Your abdominal muscles are completely relaxed.	Think about your abdominal muscles being completely relaxed.
Your chest, arms, neck, head are completely relaxed.	Think about your chest, arms, neck, head, being completely relaxed.

Muscle group tension and relaxation

Assume a comfortable, supported position on your back, on the floor, in a lounge chair, or in a recliner. Take a deep, relaxing breath, and relax your whole body. To completely relax, you may want to repeat Exercise 1.

Exercise 3: Muscle group tension and relaxation

Direction	Action
Tense your right arm.	Tense your entire right arm by straightening it. Ignore your right arm and concentrate on the feeling of relaxation in the rest of your body.

Partner checks for relaxation in all body parts except the right arm.

Release your right arm.	Release tension from your right arm.
Tense your left arm.	Tense your left arm by straightening it. Ignore your left arm and concentrate on the feeling of relaxation in the rest of your body.

Partner checks for relaxation in all body parts except the left arm.

Release your left arm.	Release all tension in your left arm.
Tense and release your right leg, then your left leg.	Tense, ignore, and release your right leg, then your left leg.
Tense and release both arms, both legs, right arm and right leg, left arm and left leg, right arm and left leg, left arm and right leg.	Tense, ignore, and release both arms, both legs, right arm and right leg, left arm and left leg, right arm and left leg, left arm and right leg.

Back and face tension and relaxation

Practice this exercise in side-lying, sitting, and standing positions. Take a deep, relaxing breath, and relax your whole body. Concentrate on how your back and face muscles feel as you tense and release them.

Exercise 4: Back and face tension and relaxation

Direction	Action
Arch your back.	Arch your back. Note spread of tension to your legs and neck.

Release your back to the count of ten.	Release your back to the count of ten. Note the gradual release of tension.
Push your back into the surface you are lying on.	Push your back into the surface you are lying on. Note the spread of tension.
Release your back to the count of ten.	Release your back to the count of ten. Note the gradual release of tension.
Tense your forehead and eyes.	Tense your forehead and eyes by frowning and squinting. Note the spread of tension.
Release your forehead and eyes to the count of ten.	Release your forehead and eyes to the count of ten. Note the gradual release of tension.
Tense your lower face.	Tense your lower face by clenching your teeth and grimacing. Note the resulting tension in your jaw and neck.
Release your lower face to the count of ten.	Gradually release tension to the count of ten.
Tense your tongue.	Press your tongue firmly against the roof of your mouth. Note the spread of tension down your throat.
Release your tongue to the count of ten.	Release your tongue to the count of ten. Note the gradual release of tension.
Completely release your whole body.	Make sure your whole body is completely relaxed.

Assume a comfortable, supported position on your back on the floor, in a lounge chair, or in a recliner. As you tense and rotate one part of your body, concentrate on keeping the rest of your body relaxed.

Motion with release

Exercise 5: Motion with release

Direction	**Action**
Tense your right hand while slowly rotating it in a circle.	Tense your right hand and gently rotate it in circles. Concentrate on keeping the rest of your body relaxed.

Partner checks for relaxation in all body parts except the moving part.

Release your right hand.	Stop the motion and release your right hand.
Tense, slowly rotate, and release your **left hand,** **right arm,** left arm, right foot, left foot, right leg, left leg.	Tense and rotate the body part as directed. Concentrate on keeping the rest of your body relaxed. Stop the motion and release as directed.
Tense and rotate your right arm and left leg.	Tense your right arm and left leg while rotating them gently in circles. Concentrate on keeping the rest of your body relaxed.

Partner checks for relaxation in all body parts except the moving parts.

Release your right arm and left leg.	Stop the motion and release your right arm and left leg.
Tense other combinations of arms, legs, feet, and hands while rotating them in a circle. Release them.	Tense and rotate the combination of body parts as directed. Concentrate on keeping the rest of your body relaxed. Stop the motion and release as directed.

Switching   Assume a comfortable, supported position on your back on the floor, in a lounge chair, or in a recliner. As you tense one muscle or muscle group and release it, learn to switch to the same muscle or muscle group on the other side of your body.

Exercise 6: Switching

Direction	**Action**
Tense your right hand.	Tense your right hand by making a fist.
Release your right hand and switch.	Release your right hand and tense your left.

Release your left hand.

Tense, release, switch, and release
arms,
shoulders,
feet,
legs.

Tense your right arm and right leg.

Release your right arm and right leg and switch.

Release your left arm and left leg.

Tense, release, switch, and release other combinations of arms, legs, hands, feet, and shoulders.

Release your left hand.

Tense, release, switch, and release as directed.

Tense your right arm and right leg. Remember to point your heel, not your toe, when you tense your legs.

Release your right arm and right leg. Tense your left arm and left leg.

Release your left arm and left leg.

Tense, release, switch, and release combinations as directed.

Patterned breathing

The Lamaze method of childbirth preparation is based on the principle of conditioned response—a learned reaction that becomes automatic through practice. The Lamaze method conditions women to respond to uterine contractions by relaxing voluntary muscles and using controlled breathing patterns. As a laboring woman concentrates on the breathing patterns, her awareness of the contraction diminishes. Although the intensity of the contraction is not altered by relaxation or the breathing patterns, a woman's perception of the intensity changes.

The Lamaze breathing patterns for labor and delivery are designed to help a laboring woman (1) relax, (2) focus her concentration, and (3) maintain an adequate supply of oxygen with a minimum expenditure of energy. The muscles that make up the uterus demand oxygen to function efficiently in labor. Lack of oxygen and glucose, and waste products of metabolism (lactic acid) in the uterine muscles can cause pain. Breath-holding or rapid, irregular breathing combined with muscle tension inhibits circulation and interferes with the delivery of oxygen and glucose to the uterus and the removal of uterine wastes. Controlled breathing, relaxation, and proper body positioning, on the other hand, promote circulation and minimize competition for the available blood supply.

During "early" labor, normal breathing in combination with total body relaxation is usually sufficient to maintain comfort. Since normal breathing requires less energy than the Lamaze breathing patterns, you should use normal breathing as long as it helps you remain comfortable during contractions. Subsequent breathing patterns use shallow breathing which helps keep the diaphragm from interfering with the upward and outward expansion of the abdomen as the uterus contracts.

When you switch to the Lamaze breathing patterns, begin and end each contraction with a deep relaxing breath by breathing in through your nose and blowing out through your mouth. These relaxing breaths remind you to relax your body completely as a contraction begins and ends. Some women find that their ability to concentrate is enhanced if they keep their eyes open and focus on a specific spot in the room, a favorite picture, or a special object. Other women find they can concentrate and relax more completely by closing their eyes.

As you practice the breathing patterns, try to breathe in a consistent rhythm. This ensures that the amount of air you inhale equals the amount of air you exhale and that the amount of oxygen and carbon dioxide in your blood remains adequate. When you upset the balance of these two gases in your circulatory system by emphasizing either inhalation or exhalation, hyperventilation results. The early symptoms of hyperventilation include light-headedness; shortness of breath; numbness; stiffness; tingling of the fingers, toes, and area around the mouth. More advanced symptoms include spasms of the face, hands, or chest. Should hyperventilation occur, you can slow down your breathing, or cup your hands over your mouth and nose and breathe until the symptoms disappear, or breathe into a paper bag, or hold your breath awhile.

Suggestions for practicing and using the breathing patterns

As you practice the Lamaze breathing patterns, keep the following suggestions in mind:

- Establish a steady, regular rhythm in each breathing pattern. Since it is natural to breathe faster during labor than in practice, it is important to keep your practice breathing slow and even.

- Practice the breathing patterns in a variety of positions—sitting, standing, lying down, on all fours—since during labor you will be varying your position frequently.

- If you are experiencing Braxton-Hicks contractions during your pregnancy, use them as an opportunity to practice the breathing patterns and active relaxation.

- Begin with practice contractions of 30 seconds in length, and progress until you can practice at least 60-second contractions. In early labor, the contractions will be shorter than 60 seconds. In the late active phase of labor they will be 60-90 seconds long and may even seem continuous as they come very close together.

- Practice the breathing patterns through several practice contractions each day. The more conscientious you are about your practice, the more conditioned you will become.

The following suggestions will be helpful as you use the breathing patterns during labor:

- In labor, begin a breathing pattern with a relaxing breath in response to the sensation that a contraction is beginning. When you feel the contraction subside, take another relaxing breath and resume normal breathing.

- Begin a new breathing pattern when the one you are currently using no longer helps you concentrate and relax during a contraction. You will be able to tell when the contractions are more intense and demand a more active, complex breathing pattern. Your partner will also recognize your need to change breathing patterns, since you will probably look more uncomfortable, tense, and restless.

- Breathing patterns during labor can be combined with effleurage, the pelvic tilt in all positions, back pressure and massage, and passive pelvic tilt.

- Use the rest time in between contractions to enhance your comfort. Walk, change your position in the chair or bed, use the bathroom, relax your body, chew ice chips.

During practice, you, the partner, can give verbal cues—"contraction begins" and "contraction ends"—to identify when to begin and end breathing patterns. Occasionally during practice you can use manual pressure instead of words to simulate the intensity of a uterine contraction. Begin a practice contraction with a firm pressure on the woman's arm or leg. Increase pressure as the contraction reaches a peak, and gradually release the pressure as the practice contraction ends. Practice the breathing patterns so you can breathe with the laboring woman should she need someone to do so for encouragement and support. Some women respond to counting or tapping with a finger to help them maintain the breathing pattern, particularly during the active phase of the first stage of labor. Help the woman identify muscle tension

The partner's role in patterned breathing

during practice and labor. A light touch on the tense area may help her relax. Verbally pace the contractions, periodically telling how many seconds have elapsed. Help the woman control hyperventilation by remaining calm yourself and giving her verbal reassurance. If necessary, set a slower rate of breathing by having her focus on you. Remember, the hospital nurses are familiar with the breathing patterns. They will support you as you assist the laboring woman.

Contractions A contraction is often described as a wave-like feeling. It is mild as it begins, grows in intensity as it reaches its peak, and tapers off as the muscles of the uterus relax. As labor progresses, the peak or most intense portion of the contraction lasts longer. In response to contractions, there are three basic Lamaze breathing patterns—slow chest-breathing, shallow chest-breathing, and pant-blow.

Slow chest-breathing Use this breathing pattern in the "early phase" of the first stage of labor when normal respiration and complete relaxation are no longer helping you to concentrate and relax. You will know when to begin this pattern of breathing because you will feel more uncomfortable and possibly restless and anxious during contractions.

It may also be helpful to use this breathing pattern during the rest periods between contractions in the later phases of labor if you still feel discomfort and/or tension after a contraction ends. This breathing pattern is also useful during medical procedures that may be performed during the birth process.

Take an initial relaxing breath in through your nose and out through

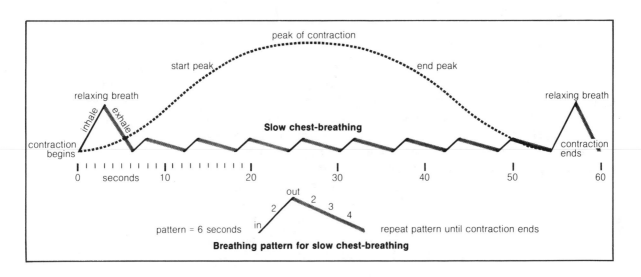

your mouth. Then breathe in through your nose for two seconds keeping your mouth closed but relaxed, and exhale through a relaxed, open mouth for four seconds. Purse your lips slightly during exhalation to ensure that you exhale the same amount of air you inhaled. Continue this breathing pattern throughout the contraction. When the contraction subsides, take a relaxing breath.

Use this breathing pattern when slow chest-breathing is no longer effective for comfort and relaxation.

Shallow chest-breathing

    Shallow chest-breathing is a quick, active one-second inhalation through your nose with your mouth closed, followed by a passive one-second exhalation through your very relaxed mouth. You will exchange the same amount of air on inhalation and exhalation at the rate of approximately 30 respirations per minute.

    As the "active phase" of labor progresses, contractions increase in intensity, length, and duration. As you use shallow chest-breathing, you will feel the need to increase the rate and decrease the depth of your breathing just a little bit as the contractions change in character. The peaks of contractions during this phase of labor last longer, and during these peaks you will probably feel the need to increase the rate of shallow chest-breathing to a half-second inhalation followed by a half-second exhalation.

    Begin the contraction with a relaxing breath and adapt shallow chest-breathing to the intensity of the contraction by breathing more quickly at the peak of the contraction. When the peak begins to ease, resume the

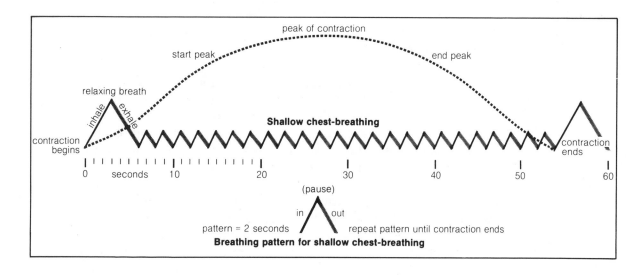

Breathing pattern for shallow chest-breathing

shallow chest-breathing pattern, or a one-second inhalation followed by a one-second exhalation.

To practice this breathing pattern, work with a 60-second contraction that builds for 15 seconds (use shallow chest-breathing), maintains a peak intensity for 30 seconds (use adapted shallow chest-breathing), and tapers off for 15 seconds (shallow chest-breathing).

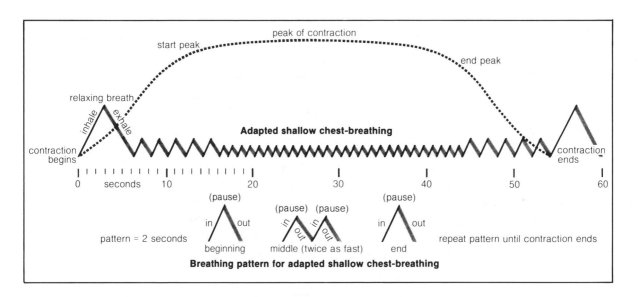

Breathing pattern for adapted shallow chest-breathing

Pant-blow breathing This breathing pattern is a series of light, shallow pants followed by a quick blow. You use it when shallow chest-breathing is no longer helping you maintain comfort and relaxation. As contractions become longer and closer together, this breathing pattern may help you to concentrate and control a premature urge to push.

Do the pant-blow pattern through your mouth. Following the initial relaxing breath, put your tongue lightly on the roof of your mouth behind your upper teeth. This position helps to warm and moisten the inhaled air in an attempt to prevent your mouth from becoming too dry. After the initial relaxing breath, take six high, shallow breaths in and out through your mouth. Breathe in a seventh time and blow steadily for one and one-half seconds as if trying to cool soup. Continue this pattern throughout the contraction, and end with a relaxing breath. The pants are approximately a half-second inhalation, a half-second exhalation.

As your urge to push intensifies or the contractions simply become stronger, change this pattern from six pants to four pants to two pants, followed by a one-and-one-half-second blow. The blow is deliberate to help control the urge to push. It is important to keep the respirations light and steady and to try to remain relaxed.

The contractions during the "late active phase" of the first stage of labor may peak from the moment they begin. Therefore, you may feel the need to eliminate the relaxing breath at the beginning of the contractions and simply begin the pattern. Continue, however, to take a relaxing breath at the end of each contraction.

The urge to push the baby out of the birth canal is a strong, natural reflex reaction to the pressure the baby's presenting part exerts on your pelvic floor as the baby descends into the birth canal. The position of the baby, your position, and whether you have received any type of anesthesia are factors that affect the urge to push or bear down. You may experience this urge as an intermittent or a continuous sensation throughout the contraction. Some women experience the urge to push too soon; some feel it at the appropriate time; and other women never feel the urge to push at all. If you experience the urge to push or bear down too soon, and if the person attending you has instructed you not to push, try the two-pant blow ("and pant and pant and blow"). If this doesn't work, try the F-blow (saying the letter "F" in rapid succession). Continue these light, rapid exhalations until the urge to push diminishes or the contraction ends. Another breathing pattern that may help is simply saying "hee who" in rapid succession until the urge to push passes or the contraction is over.

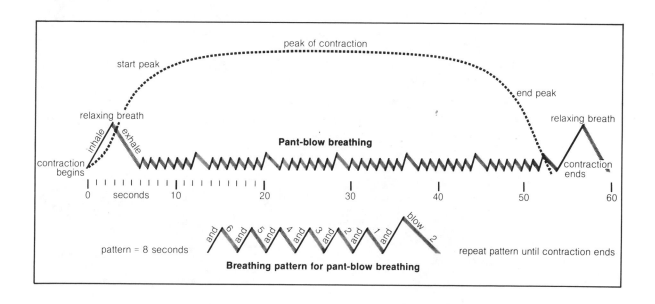

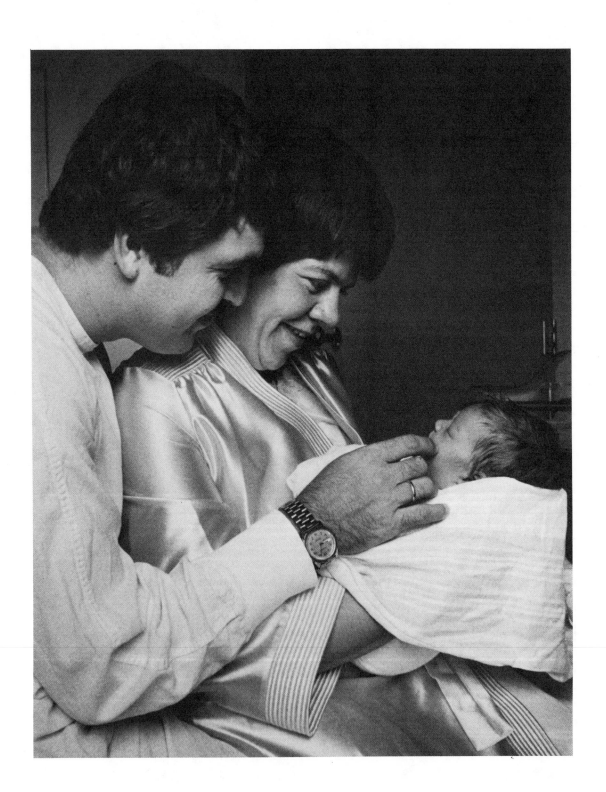

CHAPTER 6

Labor and Birth

Your childbirth partner

Anyone can be a childbirth partner—the baby's father; a relative, friend, or neighbor; a Lamaze instructor—as long as you feel mutually comfortable with each other and with the idea of partnership during childbirth. Whomever you choose, it is important for your partner to receive training in the Lamaze method, to attend classes with you, and to be available to help you practice the relaxation, breathing, and comfort techniques prior to labor. The extent of a partner's participation varies with each individual. Some women need a partner's physical support; some women need a partner's emotional support; other women need the presence of a familiar person in an unfamiliar setting. To fulfill these commitments and needs, it is helpful when your partner has a flexible schedule that allows time to practice and to go to the hospital for childbirth. Someone with a demanding job or young children, for example, may not be available at the last minute.

Relatives often volunteer as childbirth partners. They work well as long as their emotional involvement with you does not interfere with their ability to help. Women who have given birth using the Lamaze method often make helpful partners because they know how you are feeling and what you are experiencing. Some hospitals allow more than one person to accompany you. This is especially important if you are planning to include your children in the childbirth process.

When a woman chooses the baby's father as her childbirth partner, it is not unusual for the father to remain enthusiastic about his role as childbirth partner long after the baby is born. The father is, after all, a unique partner. His is a familiar face, voice, and touch in unfamiliar surroundings. He provides physical support and comfort as well as emotional support and encouragement. Since the father and mother have shared the long months of pregnancy and the changes it brings, they are the people most interested in the birth of their child. It is fitting for them to share the experience.

Lamaze class instructors encourage prospective fathers and mothers to share their concerns about pregnancy, labor, delivery, and parenthood. Group discussions enable fathers and mothers to share questions, problems, and insights about the team approach to childbirth. The childbirth team includes the mother, the father or partner, the nurses, and the mother's health care provider. The father's role on the team is vital, and he may feel apprehensive or even overwhelmed by it. Lamaze classes, however, will help him learn and practice skills for coping effectively with labor and delivery.

Whether your partner is the father or someone else, you will need to keep your partner informed of your progress during the last few weeks of pregnancy. If possible, have your partner accompany you on prenatal visits or check in with your partner after each visit to your health care provider. Together you will want to arrange

- How you can reach your partner days, nights, weekends
- When you will alert your partner
- Where you will meet, at your house or the hospital/birthing center
- How you will get to the hospital/birthing center

The partner's role during pregnancy

As a woman's childbirth partner, one of your major roles during her pregnancy is to become informed about the childbirth process. You can do this by reading this book and other books about childbirth, attending Lamaze classes, and accompanying her on prenatal health care visits. The more you know about her pregnancy, active relaxation, the breathing patterns, and comfort measures, the more you will be able to help during childbirth.

During pregnancy, you will also want to practice the breathing patterns, comfort measures, and active relaxation exercises together. Practice sessions can be a relaxing time together during pregnancy and will give you both a feeling of confidence during childbirth.

Throughout the woman's pregnancy, you can work together to identify and alleviate tension-producing situations. You can also provide moral support, encouragement, affection, and help with household routines and activities.

During the woman's labor at home and at the hospital, there are a number of specific ways you, the partner, can provide comfort, support, and reassurance:

- Remind her to rest, drink fluids, and empty her bladder. If she anticipates a cesarean delivery, remind her not to eat, since eating increases the likelihood of vomiting.

- Watch her face and limbs for signs of tension and help her relax using active relaxation. You can also suggest head rolls, shoulder shrugs, arm stretches, and a warm shower. Remember, too, the notion that "touching is worth at least 75 milligrams of Demerol an hour to ease a woman's discomfort."*

- Remind her of the breathing patterns and help her do them effectively.

- Administer comfort measures including the backrub, counterpressure, effleurage, hot washcloths on her abdomen, gentle stroking of her extremities, or whatever she finds most soothing.

- Encourage her to change positions frequently to promote circulation. You can suggest sitting, standing, leaning, pelvic tilt, side-lying, and back-lying for comfort and variety.

- Time and pace contractions for her.

- At the hospital, help interpret her needs, likes, and dislikes to hospital personnel. They may also suggest additional ways you can be helpful.

- Offer her sips of water, ice chips, lip balm, and cool cloths for her forehead, neck, and lips. If she is cold, help her put on socks and get her a blanket.

- Remember to take a break yourself. Go to the bathroom, get a snack, or just sit and rest for a few minutes. Notify your nurse when you leave so she can check on the mother more often or stay with her in your absence. You may feel more comfortable about leaving if you tell your nurse where you can be reached.

- Call a nurse to check the mother when she first experiences the urge to push. The nurse will help you help the mother into the desired pushing position. Assist and encourage her as she pushes.

- Praise and assure the mother that she is doing a fine job, especially when she feels she cannot go on. Remember, mothers anticipating a cesarean delivery need the same kind of support and encouragement.

---

*Tracy Hotchner, *Pregnancy and Childbirth,* p. 391.

The partner's role if the mother panics

Occasionally the mother may lose her ability to cope with the childbirth process. If this is the case, you may see her tossing her head from side-to-side, grasping the siderails, clenching her teeth, grimacing, gasping for breath. She may tell you, "I can't do this any more," or "You've got to do something." Here are some steps that can help her regain control:

1. Hold the mother's head between your hands. Establish eye contact and acknowledge her feelings by saying, "I am with you," or "I'll help you," or "This is really hard work," or "This must be difficult for you."

2. Tell her to release her hands, relax her face, loosen her jaw.

3. Begin breathing with her but not for the full length of the contraction, since doing so may make you light-headed and dizzy. Shift to verbal directions if she needs them—"And one and two and blow."

4. Reassure her as she grows calmer. Remind her that she is doing a good job and update her on her progress.

Remember, your presence during childbirth is important. You are a vital part of the childbirth team. At times you may feel overwhelmed, worried that you do not have all the answers, or afraid that you might do the wrong thing. These are all natural feelings. If you feel yourself starting to panic, use the bedside call button to summon hospital staff. They can provide needed relief, support, and assurance. If this is your first childbirth experience, be prepared for the fact that at times it may be more strenuous and emotional than you anticipated. Like the mother, you will have your ups and downs too.

Having a partner for cesarean delivery

Many mothers and fathers believe the method of delivering their baby should not interfere with their desire to be together during childbirth. They have shared the months of the pregnancy and want to share the birth experience, whether the baby is born vaginally or by cesarean delivery. As childbirth partner during a cesarean delivery, the father provides support, reassurance, and encouragement. He experiences his child's first moment of life and may be able to hold the baby. Neither he nor the mother can see delivery because of sterile draping. Throughout the delivery, he is seated next to the mother's head and may leave the room from time to time if he feels uncomfortable.

Whether you want the father or someone else for your childbirth partner during cesarean delivery, you will need to check with the hospital, the anesthesiologist, and your health care provider. Many hospitals permit partners to attend a cesarean delivery, but some do not. Many hospitals, however, require some sort of preparation before granting permission for a partner to be present during cesarean delivery. LCPA, other childbirth education groups, and many hospitals offer classes on cesarean births.

Some women do not choose to have a childbirth partner, and even if you plan on a partner, there may be occasions when your partner is temporarily unavailable—admitting you to the hospital, taking a break for a snack, going to the restroom—or when your partner is out of town or suddenly ill and unable to participate at all. Whatever the reason, should you find yourself without a partner for some or all of the childbirth process, the nursing staff will be supportive. To prepare yourself for the possibility of laboring without your partner, consider the following:

Having no childbirth partner

1. During Lamaze classes, make a tape of the relaxation and breathing exercises to help you practice at home.

2. Practice the relaxation exercises faithfully. Once you have developed the ability to relax, practice relaxing when you are excited or pressured. This will help you relax during your labor when excitement and tension are likely to intensify.

3. Practice the breathing techniques. Concentrate on controlling the rate. While practicing, do effleurage, self-backrub, constant back pressure (lying on your fists, or tennis balls), and pelvic tilt. Also change your position frequently. This practice in doing several things at once will help you do them simultaneously during labor.

4. When you arrive at the hospital, tell the nurses that you do not have a labor partner. Request their support.

5. During labor, call a nurse for comfort measures including ice chips, cool or warm cloths, a backrub, a bedpan, help in changing positions.

6. If you fall asleep between contractions, try slow chest-breathing between contractions to help you stay alert and in control.

7. Most hospitals allow at least one person to stay with you. If you change your mind about laboring alone, a friend or relative can be with you whether or not the person is trained in the Lamaze method. The presence of a familiar person can be very supportive.

8. If you are feeling tense and losing control, ask for a nurse who is familiar with the Lamaze method to stay with you. Also, once you experience the urge to push, a nurse will stay with you through delivery.

Labor and Birth   91

The first stage of labor: The three phases

Labor is the process in which the uterine muscles contract to propel the baby from the uterus, past the cervix, through the birth canal, and into the world. On the average, labor takes from eight to twelve hours for the first baby and about six hours for subsequent babies. Labor for every baby is different, however, and the length of labor depends on conditions beyond your control—your baby's position and size, contraction efficiency, and the cervix's ability to soften and dilate. The "late active phase," however, usually progresses more rapidly than the "early phase."

The purpose of labor is to remove the baby from the protective environment where it has grown and matured for 40 weeks. Labor begins when the uterine muscles begin to contract or tighten. As they tighten, they shorten and stretch the cervix and exert pressure on the contents of the uterus—the baby, amniotic fluid, and placenta. As a result, the cervix effaces (thins out) and dilates (opens up) so that the baby can pass into the birth canal (vagina). Continued uterine contractions and the mother's active pushing further propel the baby through the birth canal and into the world.

The labor process occurs in three stages. The first stage is the effacement and dilatation of the cervix and includes the early labor phase when the cervix effaces and dilates from zero to three centimeters (cm), the active labor phase when the cervix dilates from three to seven centimeters, and the late active labor phase, or transition, when the cervix dilates from seven to ten centimeters. The second stage is when the baby is born, and the third stage involves the expulsion of the placenta, or "afterbirth."

Preliminary signs of labor

In the weeks and days before the baby is due, a woman may experience one or more of the following feelings or changes that signal the imminent onset of labor:

- Engagement, or lightening, occurs when the baby settles into the pelvis two to four weeks before delivery. In women who have previously given birth, lightening often occurs later with the onset of labor.

- Braxton-Hicks contractions often increase and become quite regular. These contractions help tone the uterus and soften the cervix.

- Unexplained weight loss, or the leveling off of weight gain, is common during the last week of pregnancy as retained fluid is lost.

Cervix during labor and birth

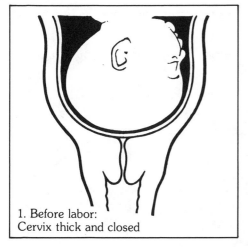

1. Before labor:
Cervix thick and closed

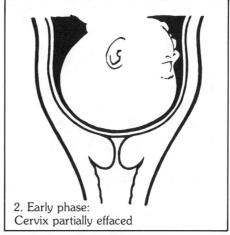

2. Early phase:
Cervix partially effaced

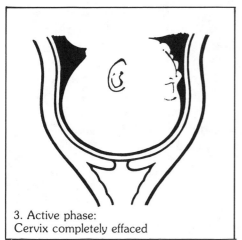

3. Active phase:
Cervix completely effaced

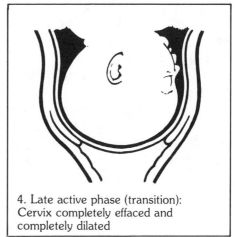

4. Late active phase (transition):
Cervix completely effaced and
completely dilated

Dilatation of the cervix during phases of labor

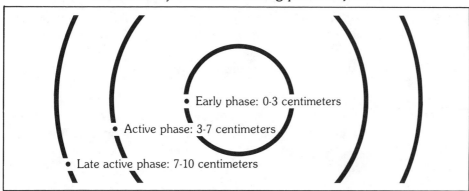

- Early phase: 0-3 centimeters
- Active phase: 3-7 centimeters
- Late active phase: 7-10 centimeters

- The nesting instinct, a spurt of energy, often occurs one or two days before delivery.

- Reduced movement of the baby is often noticeable about two days before delivery or just after lightening.

- Vaginal discharge increases, especially after a vaginal exam, intercourse, or lifting a heavy object. Do not be concerned if a little blood streaks the mucus after a vaginal exam.

- Change in bowel habits may occur.

If you think you are in labor, relax. Running around burns up needed energy. At night, try to sleep a little longer. During the day, rest or do something easy and relaxing. Use active relaxation, slow chest-breathing, and comfort measures as needed.

Eat if you feel hungry. When and how much you eat probably does not influence nausea and vomiting during labor. If you do not feel like eating, remember to drink fluids to prevent dehydration and maintain energy.

Notify your health care provider or the hospital. Your health care provider may want you to go to the office or the hospital to be checked for progress before admitting you to the hospital. Try not to be discouraged if you are sent home for a while until the contractions pick up or until you progress a little further. A vaginal exam is the only way to determine how far your cervix has effaced and dilated.

Prodromal, or "false," labor You may experience a series of contractions that feel like Braxton-Hicks contractions and continue for hours or start and stop over a period of days or weeks. Such contractions, which you will feel mainly in your abdomen, are more common after the first pregnancy. They may accomplish effacement and some dilatation, but they do not continue long enough to initiate productive labor. They may be irregular, will not occur in a predictable pattern, will have long intervals between them, and will not increase in intensity. As you change your activity or position, these contractions will usually diminish or stop.

The early labor phase The contractions of productive labor usually develop a predictable pattern over time and grow closer together and more intense. You may feel these contractions in your back, or they may start in your back and move to your abdomen. Activity such as walking stimulates these contractions, and relaxing or taking a warm shower will not make them go away. They may feel like menstrual cramps, a backache, intestinal distress, gas, or your abdomen tightening into a fist.

Early labor contractions usually increase from 20 seconds to 45 seconds in length while the interval between contractions decreases from 20 minutes to 5 minutes. Contractions can start at less than 20 minutes apart, however. During a woman's first labor it often takes six hours or more for the cervix to completely efface and dilate to three centimeters.

There is usually a "bloody show" as the contractions push out the mucous plug. This show of blood may be unreliable if you have just recently had a vaginal exam.

Be sure to contact your health care provider when you experience a gush or trickle of fluid from the vagina, which indicates that the membranes have ruptured. Note whether the fluid is clear or dark. If you are uncertain whether or not the membranes have ruptured, your health care provider may perform a nitrazine test in the office or in the labor and delivery area. During a vaginal exam, a piece of nitrazine paper is touched to the vaginal secretions. If the paper changes from yellow to dark blue, alkaline amniotic fluid is present. If the nitrazine test is inconclusive, a ferning test may be done to document ruptured membranes: the health care provider inserts a speculum into the vagina, swabs secretions from the cervical canal, and applies them to a glass slide. If the secretion is amniotic fluid, it will form a crystalline, fern-like pattern when viewed under a microscope.

If you are unable to tell whether or not your contractions are productive, call your health care provider. Your health care provider will be able to determine the productiveness of your contractions by doing a vaginal exam. Without an exam, you might assume that you are having false labor, when in fact you are fully dilated and ready to deliver.

Hospital admission

Because procedures vary from one hospital to another, take a hospital tour well in advance of your due date so that when it is time to go to the hospital, you will know where to go and what to do. During one of your prenatal visits, ask your health care provider for instructions about when you should go to the hospital once you are in labor. Generally, women expecting first babies go to the hospital when contractions have been three to five minutes apart for one hour.

When you arrive at the hospital, a hospital physician will examine you vaginally and notify your health care provider of your arrival and exam results. Based on exam results, your health care provider either admits you to the hospital or sends you home with further instructions about when to come again.

Your baby during labor and birth

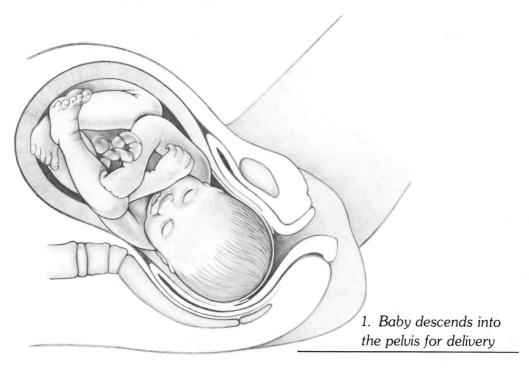

1. Baby descends into the pelvis for delivery

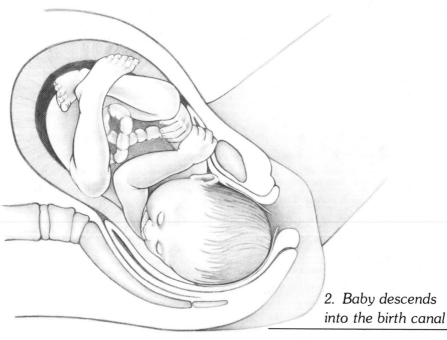

2. Baby descends into the birth canal

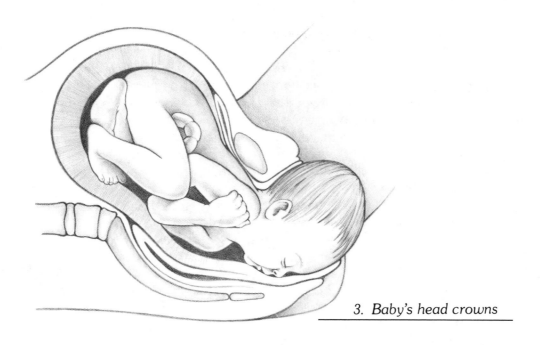

3. Baby's head crowns

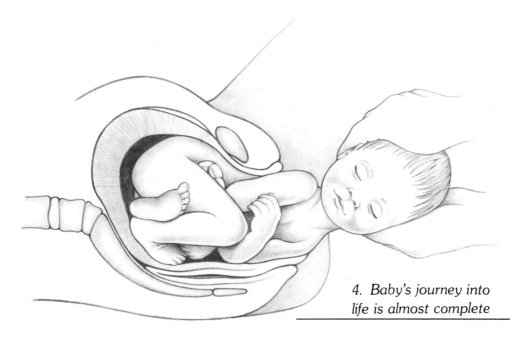

*4. Baby's journey into
life is almost complete*

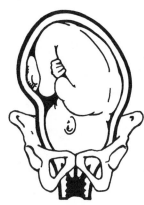

Left Occiput
Anterior Position
(LOA)

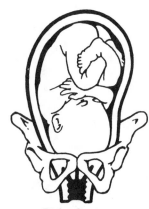

Right Occiput
Posterior Position
(ROP)

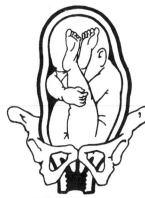

Breech Position

Once you are admitted, the hospital physician will take your health history, make a brief physical examination, and draw a blood specimen. A nurse will take your admission history, which includes questions about your name, age, occupation, number of children, religion, due date, previous pregnancies and miscarriages, past serious illnesses or operations, and allergies to foods and medications. The nurse will also ask you about your present pregnancy—what problems you have had; what your weight gain has been; when your contractions started; what the duration, frequency, and intensity of your contractions are; whether your membranes have ruptured; if you have noticed a bloody show; whether you have been recently exposed to an infectious disease; if you have a history of herpes infection or have an active herpes lesion. The nurse will take your blood pressure, temperature, pulse, and respiration and ask you for a urine specimen. You or the hospital physician may request an enema to empty your lower bowel.

Next, the nurse or hospital physician will listen to the baby's fetal heart tones (FHT, heartbeat) and check the position of the presenting part of the baby by feeling your abdomen. Most babies are positioned head down with the back part of the skull (occiput) toward the mother's abdomen (anterior) and the baby's back along the mother's left side. This is the left occiput anterior (LOA) position. If the baby's back is lying along the mother's right side, the position is right occiput anterior (ROA). If the back of the baby's head is toward the mother's spine (posterior), the baby is either in right occiput posterior (ROP) position, or left occiput posterior (LOP) position. If the baby's buttocks or feet are first, or down in the pelvic basin, the baby is in breech position.

Along with the baby's position, the nurse or hospital physician will check the baby's station, which is a measure of the lowest point of the baby's presenting part (head, buttocks, or feet) in relation to the two ischial bones in the mother's pelvis. Distance is measured in centimeters above (-) and below (+) the ischial bones.

Hospital admission procedures usually do not take more than ten minutes. Your partner may be with you or at the admissions desk signing admitting papers. During admission procedures, you may find the relaxation techniques helpful. Also since you will encounter many new people in the hospital setting, feel free to ask people who they are and what they do throughout your hospital stay.

Upon completing admission procedures, you will move to a labor room where a nurse will make you comfortable and your partner will join you after washing up and putting on a paper gown. Be sure to ask for anything you need as the hospital staff will try to answer your questions and meet your needs any way they can. The nurse will show you how to adjust the bed, give you a call light so you can reach her, and show your partner where the ice chips are. If you and your partner would like some privacy, close the labor-room door.

Periodically during early labor a nurse or physician will listen to the baby's heartbeat and examine you to determine the progress of your labor. Ask them to report their findings if they do not offer them. They will keep your own health care provider informed of your progress by phone or in person.

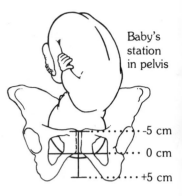

Baby's station in pelvis

-5 cm
0 cm
+5 cm

Positions for labor

Changing positions frequently as you labor may help you remain comfortable. Here are some positions to try:

- **Side-lying:** Lie on your side with your head, shoulder, and upper chest on a pillow. Straighten or slightly flex your lower leg. Bend your upper leg and put a pillow under the knee. Put a third pillow under your abdomen. Your arm position is up to you, but try putting your lower arm behind you and your upper arm on the pillow at your head.

- **Lounge chair or contour position:** Elevate the head and foot of the bed to assume a contour position. Put your arms at your sides and support each arm with a pillow. Bend your knees.

- **Sitting on the edge of the bed:** Sit at the edge of the bed with your feet supported on a chair or stool. Lean forward and rest your arms on a pillow, a bed table, or your partner.

- **Tailor-sitting:** Sit cross-legged on a bed, floor, couch, or large chair with your knees bent out and lower legs crossed or uncrossed. You can lean forward, resting your abdomen and arms on your legs, a table, a big pillow, or the foot of the hospital bed. You can also lean back against a supporting surface.

- **Standing or leaning:** Standing allows gravity to aid the descent of the baby through the pelvis. One position to try is standing with your knees slightly bent and your upper body leaning forward onto several pillows stacked on a bed or bed table. Squatting will increase the diameter of the pelvis, but be sure to hold onto something for balance. In the modified hug position, put your arms around your partner's neck and your head on your partner's shoulder. To avoid back strain, maintain pelvic tilt. Relax your legs. Have your feet apart and your hips about a foot away from your partner so that your partner can massage your back or your abdomen. Your partner may wish to lean against a wall for support. In the side-leaning position, lean at about a 30-degree angle with your shoulders against the wall. Bend and relax the leg closer to the wall. Lock the knee of your outer leg to support your weight. Your hands are free for effleurage.

The active labor phase

As labor progresses, your contractions will continue to get stronger, longer, and closer together, causing you to concentrate more on breathing patterns and active relaxation. Active labor contractions last from 45 seconds to 60 seconds and come as frequently as every four minutes. The pressure and tension of these contractions are more intense than those of early labor contractions. The cervix is dilating from three to seven centimeters. Some women use shallow chest-breathing during active labor, while others are still comfortable using slow chest-breathing. Comfort measures and emptying your bladder every hour are also helpful.

The late active labor phase, or transition

This is the most intense phase of labor, usually lasting anywhere from 20 minutes to 60 minutes, when the cervix dilates from seven to ten centimeters. The contractions reach a peak quickly and maintain a peak longer than preceding contractions. They last 60 to 90 seconds and can occur one to three minutes apart. Because of the intensity of these contractions, during them you will probably want to use adapted shallow chest-breathing or variations of the pant-blow breathing patterns, and between them, slow chest-breathing to help you relax and remain mentally alert. You may experience irritability, panic, discouragement, backache, hiccups, nausea, vomiting, trembling, leg cramps, or a hot face and cold feet. It is unlikely, however, that you will have all these symptoms of transition. Comfort measures can help. Increased rectal pressure may precede the urge to push, which may be premature. The pant-blow or F-blow breathing pattern may prevent you from pushing until your cervix is fully dilated. Depending on your cervical dilatation, the physician may have you gently push or have you pant-push when the urge to push is the strongest.

The second stage of labor: The birth process

Once your cervix is completely dilated, you can start pushing or bearing down to assist the uterine contractions as they move your baby through the birth canal. The symptoms of late active labor will subside, and you will become more aware of your surroundings between contractions, which generally last 60 seconds and are three to five minutes apart. Although it requires a lot of work, most women find pushing a relief. The urge to push varies. Some women feel an overwhelming urge, whereas others need to be told when to push. At the end of the first stage of labor, a woman having her first baby usually remains in the labor room and pushes until her vaginal opening is about the same circumference as a 50-cent piece. A woman who has previously given birth, however, usually goes directly to the delivery room at the end of the first stage of labor.

In the delivery room you may be moved from the bed or stretcher to a delivery table with leg stirrups to support your legs while you are lying or semi-sitting. A nurse will wash the area surrounding your vagina, shave the area between the vagina and rectum, and drape your body up to your chest with sterile sheets to reduce the chance of bacteria entering your birth canal. *The delivery room*

    Other people in the delivery room (in addition to your partner, your health care provider, and a nurse for the baby) may include a nurse anesthetist to insert an IV and give medications, if necessary; medical or nursing students who, with your consent, are present to observe the birth process; and a resident physician receiving specialized training by assisting your physician. In the event of cesarean birth, your pediatrician would also be present.

The sensations you feel as you push may surprise you with their force and intensity. As you push, it is important to relax the muscles of the pelvic floor. Think about opening up and letting the perineum bulge out. Warm compresses on the perineum help the tissues of the perineum relax and stretch. Massaging the area may also increase elasticity and comfort. *Pushing*

    You can push effectively in a variety of positions. The one you select will depend on how you feel, the position of your baby, your physical environment, and possibly your health care provider's preference. It is usually advisable to change positions after you spend a half hour pushing in one position without influencing the descent of the baby. Your nurse will help you assume one of the following positions for pushing:

- **Semi-sitting:** This is one of the most common pushing positions. Support your back against pillows, a wedge backrest, the adjustable back of the hospital bed, or your partner. You may also wish to pull back on your legs, use a footrest, or have your partner or a nurse hold your legs.

- **Side-lying:** This position is particularly helpful in assisting the rotation of a baby in posterior position. It helps you feel more comfortable because it removes the pressure of the baby's head from your sacrum. The side-lying position also helps delay a very rapidly descending baby. To support your upper leg, enlist your partner or the siderail of the bed.

- **Squatting:** The forces of gravity help the baby to descend through the birth canal when you push in the squatting position. You partner can help you maintain balance.

- **Kneeling and pelvic tilt:** This position may assist in the rotation of the baby during descent and relieve the pressure of the baby's head on your sacrum. You may wish to lean over the foot of the bed, a chair, or your partner's lap.

- **Back-lying:** This is the "traditional" pushing position—on your back, your feet in stirrups. You will probably use this position if you are birthing your baby in a hospital delivery room.

Breathing for pushing When you are actually experiencing the second stage of labor, your nurse or health care provider may suggest changing your breathing or your position if the baby is not descending. There are basically two ways to breathe for pushing. You may find it helpful to practice both ways and select the one that feels most comfortable.

1. For "traditional" pushing, you first relax your pelvic floor muscles. When a contraction begins, take two relaxing breaths. Take a third deep breath, contracting the upper abdominal muscles and pressing the diaphragm down towards the uterus. Round your shoulders and back and lower your chin towards your chest in a "C" curve to help direct muscular effort downward. Hold your breath for five to ten seconds by closing the back of your throat with your tongue and keeping your mouth open. A grunting sound is normal and may be helpful. Maintaining the "C" curve of your body, exhale, straighten your neck to open the airway, and inhale again to resume pushing. Repeat as often as necessary during a contraction. As the contraction ends, take two relaxing breaths, totally release all muscles and rest until the next contraction begins.

2. "Gentle" pushing involves another kind of breathing. Relax your pelvic floor muscles. When a contraction begins, take two relaxing breaths. Assume the "C" position just described and inhale. Exhale slowly and steadily through slightly pursed lips. You may hum or grunt as you exhale. When you need to inhale, do so keeping your rib cage as still as possible and continuing to contract the upper abdominal muscles. Exhale

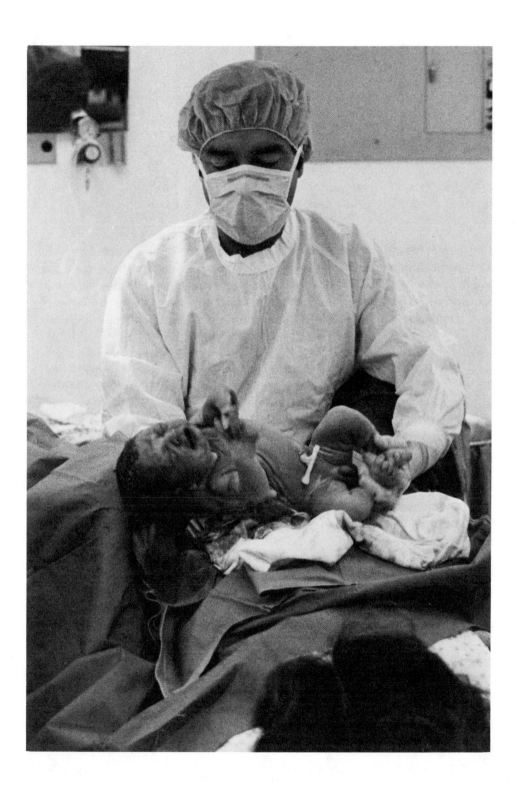

again as described. Repeat as often as necessary during a contraction. As the contraction ends, take two relaxing breaths, totally release all muscles, and rest until the next contraction begins.

When your baby begins to crown, which means that the presenting part can be seen at the vaginal opening, your health care provider will ask you to stop pushing and relax so the baby's passage through the opening is gradual and controlled. When your health care provider directs you to stop pushing, simply stop all effort, lie back, completely relax, and use a high chest pant, inhaling and exhaling through your mouth. You will feel a strong burning, stretching sensation as the baby emerges.

Unscheduled cesarean delivery

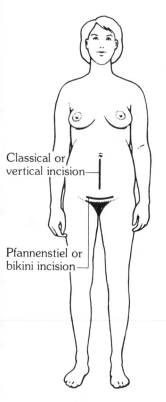

Classical or vertical incision

Pfannenstiel or bikini incision

If, at sometime during the first or second stages of labor, it appears that you are not making satisfactory progress toward a vaginal delivery or that your baby's health is endangered, your health care provider will talk with you about a cesarean delivery. A decision to perform a cesarean delivery may come as a disappointment if you were planning to deliver vaginally, or it may come as a relief that your labor is finally over. After you, your partner, your health care provider, and an anesthesiologist discuss the need for a cesarean delivery and the decision is made to go ahead with the operation, you will sign an operative permit and a nurse will ready you for the birth of your child by abdominal surgery. She will start an IV; take a blood sample in order to cross-match blood if it is needed; insert a catheter to empty your bladder; monitor your blood pressure; and shave, wash, and drape your abdomen. Continue to use active relaxation and breathing patterns throughout these procedures.

Cesarean delivery takes place in a specially equipped delivery room. After the mother has received anesthesia, the physican makes one of two types of incisions in her abdomen. An increasing number of incisions are the Pfannenstiel, or "bikini," type and run horizontally just above the pubic hairline. The other type of incision, a classical incision, runs vertically from just below the navel to the top of the pubic bone. Once the initial incision through the skin is made, the physician carefully approaches the uterus by pulling away the overlying layers of subcutaneous tissue, fatty tissue, connective tissue, and muscle. The physician controls blood loss by tying blood vessels as they are cut. The physician also retracts or draws aside the bladder. Once the uterus is visible, the physician determines the exact position of the baby and makes the incision into the uterine muscle. Whether the skin incision was horizontal or vertical, most uterine incisions run horizontally through the thin, lower portion of the uterus situated directly above the cervix. If the membranes are still intact, the physician ruptures them and delivers the

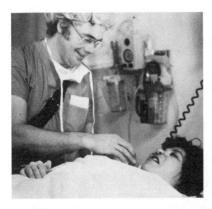
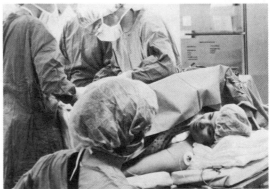

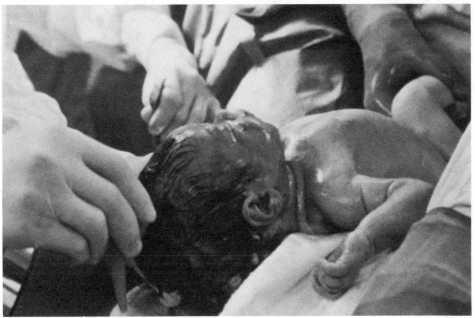

baby. Delivery takes between 10 and 15 minutes and may be manual, or the physician may use forceps especially designed for cesarean delivery. After the birth, a pediatrician usually supervises the baby's care while the physician removes the placenta through the abdominal incision and repairs the layers of tissue. Closing the incision takes from 45 minutes to an hour. Each layer of tissue is repaired separately with absorbable sutures. The final skin closure may be made with sutures or staples which are usually removed four or five days after the birth. Finally, a nurse cleanses and covers the abdomen with a sterile bandage and the new mother is wheeled to the recovery room.

The third stage of labor: The delivery of the placenta

If you give birth vaginally, your uterus will rest after your baby is born. Then it will undergo a series of rhythmical contractions to separate the placenta from the uterine wall and expel it. Expulsion of the placenta, or afterbirth, occurs from one to 20 minutes after the birth of the baby. Your physician will examine your cervix and vagina for tears or abrasions, and your placenta to be sure it is intact. Your physician may also manually examine your uterine cavity. If this is uncomfortable, slow chest-breathing or pant-blow breathing may help. After this examination, you will receive an oxytocic (contraction inducing) medication, oxytocin or ergonovine, to help the uterus remain fully contracted, closing off blood vessels in the uterine lining to prevent excessive bleeding. Some women experience chills and shaking after they expel the placenta. A warm blanket may help, along with relaxing your legs, since trying to hold still only aggravates the problem. Usually the chills and shakes pass within an hour.

After the examination of the uterus and placenta, your physician will repair the episiotomy (an incision between the vaginal opening and the anus to ease delivery) if one was performed. Each layer of tissue is repaired with absorbable sutures so there are no stitches to remove at a later time. This procedure usually takes 15 to 30 minutes, depending on the extent of the incision. When the repair is completed, a nurse will wash your perineal area, remove your legs from the stirrups, and fit you with a sanitary belt and pad to absorb the bloody vaginal discharge called lochia. (This discharge of blood, mucus, and tissue usually continues for three to eight weeks after delivery.) If you have delivered in your labor or birthing bed, you will recover in the same bed. Otherwise you will be moved from the delivery table and wheeled to the recovery room.

The baby's care in the delivery room

As soon as your baby's head is delivered, your health care provider will suction mucus from the baby's mouth and nose with a soft rubber bulb syringe to clear the airway. Usually a baby begins to cry shortly after the rest of the body is delivered. With this first cry, the lungs begin to function and the baby is no longer dependent on the oxygen the mother supplied through the umbilical cord. Before beginning to breathe unassisted, a baby may have a blue or grey color. After breathing is established, the baby begins to "pink up," although the hands and feet

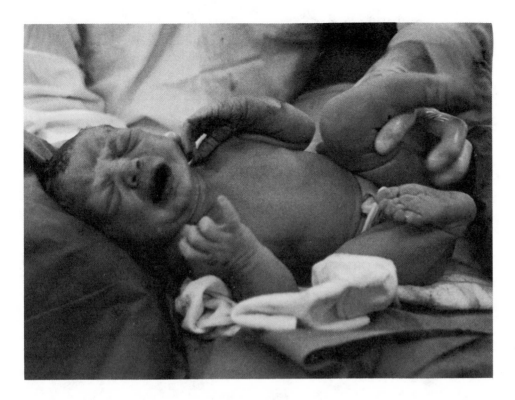

may remain blue, since the circulatory system is immature. Your health care provider may place your baby on your abdomen while clamping and cutting the umbilical cord. In some hospitals, fathers have the opportunity to cut the cord. (Ask your health care provider about this option.) You may also be able to breast feed your baby at this time.

Because a newborn's temperature often drops during the first two hours of life, a nurse will put your baby in a warming bed where she will watch your baby for physical abnormalities and breathing difficulties. She will fit you and your baby with matching identification bracelets, and within an hour after birth (in most states), will administer medication to protect the baby's eyes. (This is usually silver nitrate unless you specify tetracycline or erythromycin. See Chapter 4 for details.)

Twice, once at one minute after birth and again at five minutes after birth, a nurse will give your baby an Apgar Score. The Apgar Score is a quick and easy method of assessing a baby's heart rate, breathing, color, reflex response, and muscle tone. Your baby will receive zero, one, or two points for each of the five categories. A score of less than six points may indicate the need for special observation and care, in which case your baby may be taken directly to the newborn nursery. It is important to remember that the Apgar Score is an indication of how your baby is handling the immediate transition to life outside the uterus and has no prognostic value for your baby's future intelligence, beauty, strength, or health.

Apgar scoring chart

SIGN	0	1	2
HEART RATE	Absent	Slow (below 100)	Over 100
RESPIRATORY EFFORT	Absent	Weak cry, hypoventilation	Good strong cry
MUSCLE TONE	Limp	Some flexion of extremities	Well flexed
REFLEX RESPONSE 1. Response to catheter in nostril (tested after oropharynx is clear)	No response	Grimace	Cough or sneeze
2. Tangential foot slap	No response	Grimace	Cry and withdrawal of foot
COLOR	Blue, pale	Body pink, extremities blue	Completely pink

Ross Laboratories, Columbus, Ohio.

If there are no apparent problems, your baby will stay with you in the delivery room until you both go to the recovery room where you can nurse your baby if you have not already done so. How much time you spend together in the recovery room depends on a number of factors. A nurse will keep track of your pulse, blood pressure, and respiration, and check the condition of your uterus and episiotomy (if you had one). She will also encourage you to rest and relax. From the recovery room you

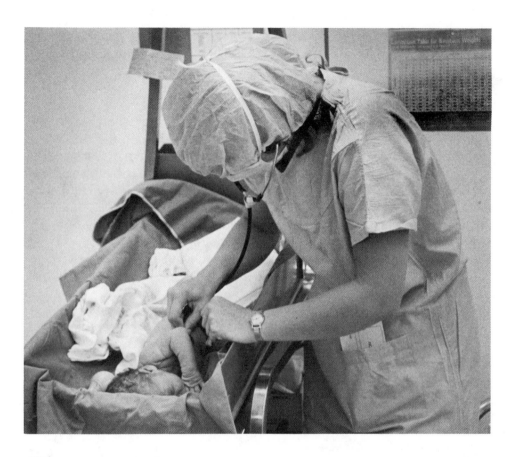

will go to a room in the postpartum unit of the hospital, and your baby will go to the newborn nursery. If, however, you have chosen early discharge, some hospitals allow you to remain in the recovery room until you are discharged.

Variations in labor and birth

Malpresentation is when the baby is not in head down (vertex) position. Vaginal delivery may be possible if the malpresentation involves posterior or breech position.

Vaginal delivery with malpresentation

A posterior presentation occurs if the baby turns the back of its head instead of its face towards the mother's spine when rotating to descend through the pelvis. The symptoms of posterior presentation are (1) a backache very low in the back and sometimes in the thighs with perhaps little or no abdominal discomfort; (2) irregular contractions varying in rate and/or intensity, especially when you are dilated between three and six centimeters; (3) slow progress early in labor; (4) restlessness, lack of confidence, and difficulty relaxing; and (5) a longer pushing period if the baby does not rotate in late active labor.

If you are experiencing the symptoms of posterior presentation, use labor positions that favor the rotation of the baby—lying on the side opposite the baby's back; kneeling, on all fours; standing or kneeling with your arms resting on a pillow or your partner; leaning your back against a fist, a tennis ball, or a hard bolster. Change your position every half hour and avoid lying on your back. During contractions, try pelvic tilt either standing or kneeling, on all fours. Pelvic tilting slowly and steadily during contractions facilitates the rotation of the baby's head away from your spine. Other comfort measures include back rubs, passive pelvic tilt, a warm or cold cloth on the lower back, effleurage, and plenty of emotional support.

Breech presentation occurs when the baby's feet or buttocks settle into the mother's pelvic basin so that during delivery the presenting part of the baby is the buttocks or legs rather than the head. Breech labor is sometimes longer because of inefficient contractions and because the buttocks and feet are not as effective in dilating or pushing as the baby's head would be. Breech presentation usually causes low backache and occurs in approximately three to four percent of all deliveries. If your baby is in breech position, there is a greater chance that you will give birth by cesarean delivery.

Emergency childbirth
In some cases the birth process progresses so rapidly that delivery occurs at home, on the way to the hospital, or in some other emergency setting without the help of medical personnel. The mother and/or the person assisting the mother should use the following procedures:

1. The mother should lie down to deliver. As the baby's head descends into the birth canal, the mother often has a sensation which she interprets as the urge to have a bowel movement. She should not go to the bathroom if delivery is imminent. She should not deliver standing over a tub or toilet.

2. Allow the baby's head to emerge slowly. The mother should not push her baby out. Pushing may tear the perineal tissue and cause undue stress to the baby. To prevent pushing, the mother should pant-blow. As the baby's head bulges the perineum, an assistant can apply gentle pressure, using a towel between hands and the perineum.

3. Do not attempt to pull the baby during delivery. The head will turn to the side, and the delivery will be spontaneous. If the cord is looped around the baby's neck, carefully loosen it by placing a finger between the baby's neck and cord. Slip the loop over the baby's shoulders as they descend. The baby will slide through the loop. Do not pull on the cord. If the membranes have not ruptured, scratch them with a sharp instrument.

4. Immediately free the baby's mouth and throat of secretions. Gently squeeze the baby's cheeks and wipe the mouth with a sterile or clean cloth. If a bulb syringe is available, gently suction the baby's mouth and nose.

5. Wrap the baby. The baby should be wrapped quickly after the birth, because the baby's temperature will drop rapidly.

6. Allow the placenta to expel itself. Do not pull on the cord to remove the placenta.

7. Keep the uterus contracted. This prevents excessive postpartum bleeding. Gently massage the mother's abdomen after the delivery of the placenta. If the baby won't nurse, stimulate the breasts manually to aid uterine contraction.

8. Take proper care of the umbilical cord. If delivery occurs in the car or if medical help will be given soon, leave the cord intact. If help will not be available for a long time, tie the cord, using two clean shoelaces. Place the first tie about two inches from the baby's navel and the second tie a little farther away. Cut between the two ties using sterilized scissors or a sterilized knife. (Sterilize by boiling for 20 minutes.)

9. Save the placenta. If you are on the way to the hospital, leave the cord and placenta attached to the baby. If the cord has been cut, save the placenta so that medical personnel can check to see that the entire placenta has been expelled.

Indicators for a cesarean delivery

Greatly improved medical, surgical, and monitoring procedures account for the increasing number of cesarean deliveries. A health care provider considers many factors and conditions when making the decision to deliver a baby in this manner. Some conditions are not by themselves reason enough for a cesarean delivery. Knowing the common indicators, however, will aid your understanding of your own birth experience, should your health care provider advise a cesarean delivery.

Cephalo-pelvic disproportion (CPD), the most easily understood indicator, occurs when the baby's head does not fit the mother's pelvis. Either the baby is very large or the mother has a small pelvic structure, although she may not be a small woman. Even when CPD is suspected prior to labor, the health care provider usually gives the woman a trial of labor. This closely monitored labor permits more accurate evaluation of the capacity of the birth canal and the change of the baby's head due to molding. While cesarean delivery is safer now, it still involves more risk and a longer recovery period than a vaginal birth. Therefore, if a vaginal delivery is possible, health care providers encourage it.

Toxemia of pregnancy is a condition in which a woman has elevated blood pressure, protein in her urine (indicating kidney involvement), and excessive swelling. While the health care provider can treat the mother's symptoms fairly well, it sometimes is advisable to deliver the baby prior to term. At this time the uterus is often unfavorable to induction of labor, and a cesarean delivery must be performed. Delivery improves the woman's condition quickly.

Dysfunctional labor occurs when the uterus does not contract effectively enough to cause dilatation of the cervix. Although factors such as the position of the baby or cephalo-pelvic disproportion may result in dysfunctional labor, the cause cannot always be identified, and a health care provider may decide to deliver the baby by cesarean.

Diabetes in the pregnant woman usually results in a larger-than-normal baby and, consequently, a difficult labor and delivery with an increased possibility of intrauterine fetal death. As a result, birth prior to term is advisable, either vaginally, if labor can be induced, or by cesarean delivery.

Placenta previa occurs when the placenta either partially or completely covers the cervix. Cesarean delivery is advisable, since if vaginal delivery were to occur, the placenta would be delivered before the baby, cutting off the baby's oxygen supply and creating an increased chance of maternal bleeding.

Placenta abruptio occurs when the placenta separates from the uterine wall. This cuts off the baby's oxygen supply and calls for an immediate cesarean delivery.

Rh incompatibility now occurs less frequently since the introduction of the drug RhoGAM. RhoGAM is given by injection to an Rh negative mother following delivery of an Rh positive infant. It provides protection during the next pregnancy by preventing the woman from producing her own permanent Rh antibodies. In cases where a mother has produced her own permanent Rh antibodies, a subsequent baby can suffer destruction of the red blood cells. If problems are suspected during pregnancy, the health care provider can check the mother's blood for antibody formation or do amniocentesis, which will give an accurate picture of fetal Rh sensitization. These tests sometimes indicate the need for immediate cesarean delivery.

There are a number of possible malpresentations that make cesarean delivery preferable. These include the transverse (lying sideways), frank breech (buttocks first), or footling breech (one or both feet coming first) presentations. The presenting part of the baby might also be the brow, a shoulder, a hand, or the face. It is impossible for the baby to be delivered vaginally in a transverse position. A baby in the breech (frank or footling) position, particularly if it is the first baby, is frequently delivered by cesarean. The problem with a breech baby is that the head, which is the largest part of the baby, is the last part to deliver and has no opportunity to mold, allowing it to fit through the birth canal.

The situation of a prolapsed cord occurs when the umbilical cord presents itself before the baby. In a vaginal birth, this would cause the baby's blood supply to be cut off because of the pressure of the baby against the cord.

Fetal distress indicated by slow or irregular fetal heart tones or heart rate, occurs when the baby's circulation is interrupted, decreasing the amount of oxygen reaching the baby. Sometimes the cause of fetal distress is apparent—a prolapsed cord. Sometimes the cause is discovered at delivery—the cord wrapped around the baby's neck. Sometimes, however, the cause of fetal distress remains unclear. Depending on the circumstances, the health care provider may feel it is safer to intervene with cesarean delivery than to wait for a vaginal delivery.

Other indicators for cesarean delivery include maternal heart disease, hypertension, or active genital herpes; postmature labor; a multiple birth; and prolonged rupture of the membranes. Your health care provider is the best source of information about these conditions. It is important to discuss together any questions or concerns you may have about the possibility of cesarean delivery.

A previous cesarean delivery is the most common indicator. Although it very seldom occurs, uterine scar tissue from a previous cesarean delivery could rupture during a subsequent vaginal birth, presenting a surgical emergency.

Vaginal birth In 1916, Dr. E. B. Craigin stated, "Once a cesarean, always a cesarean,"
after cesarean and until very recently, this has been the practice in the United States.
(VBAC) Some physicians are now willing, however, to consider the option of
vaginal birth after cesarean, commonly known as VBAC (pronounced
vee-back). These physicians believe that approximately 65 percent of all
cesarean mothers can deliver vaginally in a subsequent pregnancy.

Women consider a VBAC for a number of reasons. A VBAC
avoids the risks and inconveniences of major surgery involved in a
cesarean: the possibility of infection, gas pains, hemorrhaging, incision
pain; the side effects of anesthesia on mother and baby; a longer
hospital stay; a longer recovery period. A VBAC is 35 to 40 percent
less expensive than a cesarean delivery, which involves operating fees,
anesthesia fees, and the cost of a longer hospital stay. For some
women, a VBAC is important emotionally because they want to participate fully in labor and delivery, and they want to hold and nurse their
babies in the delivery room.

Whether or not you are a candidate for a VBAC depends on a
number of factors. It is important that the reason for your previous
cesarean delivery—placenta previa, fetal distress, malpresentation—does
not apply to the current pregnancy. During your previous cesarean
delivery you must have had a horizontal incision in your uterus. A
horizontal uterine incision minimizes the chance of uterine rupture, the
greatest risk of a VBAC, whereas a vertical uterine incision increases the
chance of uterine rupture. (Remember, your abdominal incision may differ
from your uterine incision.) Also, having had a previous vaginal birth in
addition to your cesarean increases the likelihood of VBAC.

If you are interested in a VBAC, you will want to select a physician
who supports this method of delivery. Your physician must have access
to your obstetrical records. These records must describe indicators for
your previous cesarean, the type of uterine incision used, and the
course of your postpartum recovery, since a postpartum infection
increases the risk of uterine rupture in a subsequent pregnancy. You
will also need to deliver in a hospital where an emergency cesarean can
be performed. The hospital must have an operating room available,
immediate anesthesia coverage, a 24-hour blood bank, and fetal monitoring equipment.

Things you can do to prepare for possible VBAC include maintaining
excellent health during your pregnancy, educating yourself about VBAC,
and attending childbirth preparation classes. As your pregnancy

progresses, your physician will keep track of the estimated size of your baby along with your baby's position, since a vertex presentation is most favorable for a VBAC. When you go into labor, your physician will look for normal progression of labor, generally a criteria for a VBAC. No matter how favorable things look, however, you must also prepare yourself for the possibility of a repeat cesarean, since the particular course of labor and delivery cannot be predicted.

When you are scheduled ahead of time for a cesarean delivery, you will be admitted to the hospital either the day before your delivery or the day of your delivery. Members of the nursing staff will orient you and answer your questions. They will take your vital signs including your blood pressure, temperature, pulse, and respiration rate. A nurse will take a brief history and so will a resident who will also perform a physical examination. Later, someone will draw a routine blood sample and send it to the blood bank for matching blood should it be needed. The anesthesiologist will discuss possible methods of anesthesia and have you sign permission slips for both the administration of anesthesia and the operation. A chest x-ray may be taken at this time, although many hospitals have discontinued the routine use of x-rays, since they may harm the baby and the mother.

Scheduled cesarean delivery

    Some hospitals conduct preadmission testing a day or so before admission, allowing you to remain at home until the day of your delivery. If, however, you are admitted the day before your delivery, that evening you will take a shower with an antibacterial soap and a nurse will shave your abdomen. Although you may not eat or drink anything after midnight, you may request a sleeping pill, the effects of which will have worn off by the time of your delivery. In most hospitals you may also have visitors.

    The next morning, about a half hour before delivery, you will take an antacid to buffer the acid in your stomach. You will then be transferred to the delivery room on a stretcher and helped onto the delivery table. A nurse will start an IV to provide hydration during and after the delivery, medications, blood if necessary, and general anesthesia if necessary. She will also insert a catheter into the bladder to keep it empty during surgery, to promote postoperative comfort, and to allow the monitoring of urine output. After this, your baby will be delivered as previously described.

Birth experiences: Vaginal and cesarean deliveries

The following birth experiences were written by Lamaze-trained mothers and one father shortly after their children were born. Each birth is unique. Elaine was born after a long prodromal labor. Linda arrived by cesarean delivery. Melissa almost did not make it to the hospital, and Kelly did not. She was born at home in the family room. Richard was born in a hospital birthing room, and Brian's father tells about his cesarean delivery. (Although the experiences described are real, the names and pictures in this section, and in Chapter 7, are for illustration only.)

Elaine is born

The nurse felt my abdomen during a contraction and patiently said if I stayed now (at the hospital) I would be there all day.

It is hard to express our sense of anticipation, joy, anxiety, and fear when we began Lamaze classes. We were expecting our second child, but this was our first Lamaze training. Our daughter, now five years old, had been born two months prematurely before our Lamaze classes had even started. This time we scheduled Lamaze classes a little earlier than usual in the pregnancy.

The experience with our first child had two major effects on us. The first effect was almost a feeling of celebration as I entered my last eight weeks of pregnancy with the knowledge that a baby born during this time has a good chance of survival. This feeling, however, was coupled with the uneasy feeling that "the day" could be any day after the end of the seventh month. While our Lamaze classes lasted, my spirits were high, but after the classes were over, time seemed to drag by, even though I was still feeling well and working full time.

The second effect of our first child's early birth was a feeling of fear upon hearing from both our Lamaze instructor and my doctor that, even with a full-term pregnancy, I should not expect a hard labor. This scared me because I hadn't known that I was in labor at all the first time around until the doctor checked me at four centimeters, and the baby had been born less than four hours later. I had been given an epidural block (regional anesthetic). Now I found myself facing this birth with almost no idea of what labor was like except that for me the early stages might be hard to detect and progress would be rapid.

On Friday at 3:30 a.m. I awoke feeling mild abdominal cramps that continued irregularly throughout the night. Their intensity was just enough to make me restless but not enough to keep me awake. In the morning they were accompanied by mild diarrhea as though I had a mild case of the flu. Since I had no other "flu" symptoms, I was incredibly excited—sure that this must be effacement. I waited for the contractions to increase in regularity and intensity and eagerly watched for the bloody show, but instead, around 11:30 a.m., the cramps stopped. I felt terribly disappointed, but since my "flu" also disappeared that morning, I felt that my interpretation of the signs had been correct.

On Thursday almost a week later, I found the show on my early morning trip to the bathroom, and this time it was unmistakable. My spirits soared, and I called to Hank, still in bed, "Guess you don't have to go to work today." I was scatterbrained and giggly. Hank went to work after all, and after several phone calls to my neighbor who would look after our daughter when the time arrived, I decided on staying home instead of driving to work. But except for a possible twinge or two, there were no more contractions. After a call to the doctor, my soaring spirits were on the floor. The nurses said labor could be weeks after the show and that I had probably just been experiencing Braxton-Hicks contractions the week before. Lamaze helped me out this time. I knew what I had before were not Braxton-Hicks contractions. The next day, Friday, at my regular doctor's appointment I was completely effaced and slightly dilated. I could go into labor anytime—that day or in another week!

Friday night I was restless again with slight involuntary urination, which made me wonder if the amniotic fluids were leaking. Saturday morning at 6:45 a.m., I again found a fair amount of blood after urinating. Since I knew the mucous plug was gone, I became frightened about the welfare of the baby, called the doctor, and went to the hospital to be checked. Before reaching the hospital, I began to notice contractions, but they were so mild it was difficult to time their spacing or duration. At 8:00 a.m. the resident found I was dilated to three centimeters, but the contractions were so mild that my doctor sent me out to walk around for an hour to "get things going." I was reassured, however, that the bleeding came from the dilatation of the cervix, not the baby, and that the fetal heart tones were still good.

Hank and I reparked the car and took a leisurely walk back to the hospital. While Hank went to the cafeteria for breakfast, I paced. The contractions were 30-60 seconds in duration and about four to five minutes apart, but I did not need any breathing technique to control them.

My hour was up, so I went back to the fathers' waiting room to be taken to the prep room to be checked. The delivery section was so busy, however, that I was asked to wait a little longer. I continued to pace in the fathers' waiting room, joking with Hank and the cleaning staff. The contractions were about the same strength but occasionally came at three-minute intervals. After another hour had passed, I thought I had better be checked again. The nurse felt my abdomen during a contraction and patiently said that if I stayed now I would be there all day. When the resident checked me, however, he said with no hesitation, "She must be admitted." I was dilated five centimeters.

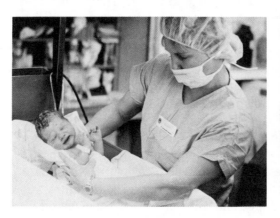 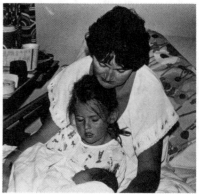

There was no time for an enema. The resident ruptured my bag of waters and immediately the strength of the contractions increased. I had to relax and use the slow chest-breathing. By now it was about 10:00 a.m. It seemed like forever before Hank joined me. (It actually was only a few minutes, even though the hospital had lost our preadmitting forms.) Shortly after, we both settled down to work in the labor room.

The contractions were much stronger now, lasting 60-75 seconds and coming two minutes apart. I had shifted to shallow chest-breathing and was tailor-sitting while Hank gave me back rubs between contractions and paced me during contractions. His pacing and presence were essential. At 11:00 a.m. the nurse checked me. I was still dilated five centimeters. I remember thinking, "A plateau. Well so much for quick labor. I must settle in for a long stay." Hank got me some ice and kept slipping it into my mouth. The cool ice felt great.

During the next hour, I should have recognized the signs of transition. The contractions were no longer regular in length or intensity, often lasting a minute and a half, or two minutes, and starting almost immediately again at full intensity with no build-up. Tailor-sitting was no longer comfortable for my back, but I had no time to change positions, as that would break my concentration. Effleurage on the upper part of my thighs helped tremendously, but when Hank tried to rub my back, I nearly jumped off the bed in reaction to his touch.

I felt a low pressure as though I had to move my bowels, but I could relax and did not feel an overriding urge to push. I used shallow chest-breathing and adapted shallow chest-breathing. Since the pressure on my bowel was especially confusing, I insisted on being checked. This was the hardest time. Contractions continued during the pelvic exam and were hard to manage. Then the nurse said, quite amazed, "She's just got the rim!" I knew that meant I was close, but I didn't know whether it meant to push or pant. I tried to ask, but in the process started to hyper-ventilate. Finally, the nurse said to try one push as they wheeled me to delivery and rushed Hank out to gown. I heard them say that with one more push the baby would crown.

The delivery room was a mad house with the draping and positioning of my legs. Hank wasn't back yet. I was afraid he would miss seeing the baby born. They paged him to hurry, and I relaxed again when he was at my head. I was given a local, which I didn't feel, and the episiotomy, and someone was trying to get me to hold my arm still to insert an IV with glucose and oxytocin.

Then I was told to push. I took the two cleansing breaths and pushed, holding onto the delivery table handles. That was a mistake. It put all the push into my arms and legs and did nothing to move the baby. The doctor pressed his fingers on my bowel. By relaxing my arms and thinking, "Okay, bowel movement or not, that's where I push," I got it right. I had to be told to breathe. I felt as though I could push forever, although Hank said I was turning blue.

Once the baby's head was born, the next push slipped her body out, and her feet were already kicking as she left the birth canal. I heard her cry and there she was on my abdomen. Elaine was born at 12:38 p.m. She was beautiful with her egg-shaped head, bluish-tinged fingers and toes, and lots of dark hair still wet and matted with a little blood.

The placenta was delivered with no trouble, and then the episiotomy was repaired. While they were checking her, I heard from behind me amidst her cries, "She's got a temper." Then came the glorious moment when she was placed first in Hank's arms, as I was helped off the delivery table, and then into mine. I had planned to nurse her at that point, but she had quite a bit of mucus, so I agreed it would be better to wait.

How did we feel? Exhilarated! First I was famished in recovery, then very tired, and oh, so happy. Although I trembled throughout recovery, I was also amazed at how good I felt. The kneading of my abdomen in recovery was uncomfortable, but I still felt great. I was ready and eager to begin nursing Elaine as soon as I was settled in a room. Now, with rooming-in, I also have her with me during the day to bathe and change and feed. It took a while; a couple false starts; a patient, reassuring husband; and a few tears before I could remain calm in the face of Elaine's screams at diaper changing, but gradually we are learning to know each other. It seems impossible that she became an independent member of our family just two days ago.

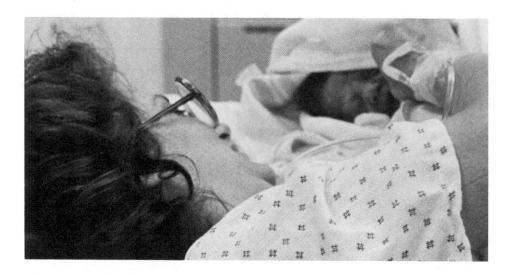

Linda is born

Her little foot had ruptured my membrane and was hanging through the cervix. The doctor didn't hesitate for a minute to tell us we would have a cesarean.

I recall our Lamaze instructor saying that, statistically speaking, one of us would have a cesarean delivery. I don't remember much else that was said concerning cesareans, because I was quite certain that I would not be the one—but I was. Four days before my due date, my doctor told me that I had already dilated one to two centimeters and that the baby was moving into position, so I assumed the baby would be born any day. We packed an elaborate "Lamaze bag" and waited anxiously.

Three days after my due date, my doctor told me that the baby had turned into breech position. It was very unusual, he said, for a baby to turn so late in a pregnancy and equally unusual for it to turn back to the normal position. They tested to see how movable the baby was and found that it wasn't very movable. Although the doctor told us to prepare ourselves for the possibility of a cesarean delivery, he also said that in our case things still looked favorable for vaginal delivery. The baby was fairly small. It was in the frank beech position (buttocks down and legs folded against the body), and my pelvic bone structure was ample. Since he also told us that breech babies are frequently late, we no longer waited anxiously, but we went about our business as if the baby weren't due for another month. (By this time I was beginning to feel that my packed suitcase was a permanent fixture in the bedroom. I checked for cobwebs when I cleaned!)

One Monday two weeks later, at about 10:00 p.m., I was in the midst of a sewing project when my water broke. I was sitting and didn't know what to expect when I stood. What I had was a steady flow, nothing like the sudden, enormous outpouring I had imagined. It was slightly pink, so I knew it was time to inform the doctor. He told us to come to the hospital, even though there was no hint of contractions.

When we arrived at the hospital around 10:30 p.m., I was examined by a resident who said the baby was still breech. He said that my doctor had ordered an x-ray to determine the baby's exact position. Meanwhile, I was given an IV and catheterized.

When my doctor arrived at about 11:00 p.m., he cancelled the x-ray because he could see the baby's foot. Her little foot had ruptured my membranes and was hanging through the cervix. He didn't hesitate for a minute to tell us that we would have a cesarean. David joined me in the labor room for 45 minutes before I was taken to surgery. David and I were a little disappointed that we weren't going to be together through the delivery, but our utmost concern was having a healthy baby. We were extremely excited that we were finally going to have the baby—however we had to have it! Our doctor talked with us about our concerns, and at 11:45 p.m. I left David and was wheeled to surgery. A nice new medical student kept David company and shared his "Lamaze sandwiches" while I was in surgery.

All I can say is that my cesarean delivery was a pleasant, wonderful experience. I had a spinal block (regional anesthetic), so I was alert throughout. Since I had not labored, I was rested and delivered under optimum conditions. I chatted with the anesthetist, who comforted me throughout surgery. When the doctor announced, "It's a girl, and she looks fine!" I was elated beyond words. Then I heard her cry, and in an instant, there she was next to me in the warming tray. Five minutes later I touched and kissed her, and right after, David got to hold her. I stayed in a surgical recovery room for an hour, and by 2:30 a.m. David and I were back together again in a recovery room. He kept dashing out to the nursery and back to tell me how Linda looked, since I really hadn't seen her for a very long time. We both saw her together when I fed her at 9:00 a.m.

My discomfort came in the next couple of days when I had to move, but I was so "high" from having the baby that I hardly noticed. All in all, I don't really feel that I had a difficult delivery, just a different delivery. I have a four- to five-inch horizontal scar just along a line where my pubic hair is growing back. I doubt the scar will show when my hair grows in completely, even when I'm wearing the skimpiest of clothes.

We both really feel that we shared the total childbirth experience, thanks to our preparedness through the Lamaze classes. David was involved throughout my pregnancy, and we weren't really disappointed that we were separated for an hour and fifteen minutes. Our goal was to work together to support one another in delivering a healthy baby. We accomplished this beautifully!

Melissa is born

As we bundled ourselves into the van and headed for the hospital, the weather was far from favorable. There was ice on the road and snow swirled in front of us as we drove. I found a focus and kept up the breathing.

The early part of the first stage of my labor must have begun early Thursday morning when I awoke with some gastric discomfort and minor intestinal cramps. I could feel my uterus contracting once in a while in what I thought were Braxton-Hicks contractions. I had a full, busy day at work during which the "cramps" continued intermittently. They were never painful but made me restless, so I moved around in my chair, which seemed to help.

That night I took a bath and went to bed early, still feeling as if I had the flu which was upsetting my intestinal tract and causing diarrhea and cramping. When I had a bloody show at about 10:00 p.m., I began to suspect that this might be the beginning of labor. I was somewhat alarmed, since my due date was still six weeks away. I called my doctor. The day before, during a prenatal visit, he had predicted that the baby might come as much as three weeks early. When I told him about the bloody show, he guessed that I might be starting to labor and that the baby would be born sometime in the next few days. Little did any of us know how wrong he would be!

At 10:30 p.m., I coughed, and with quite a memorable "pop," the water broke. From then on, everything began to happen fast! I lay on the

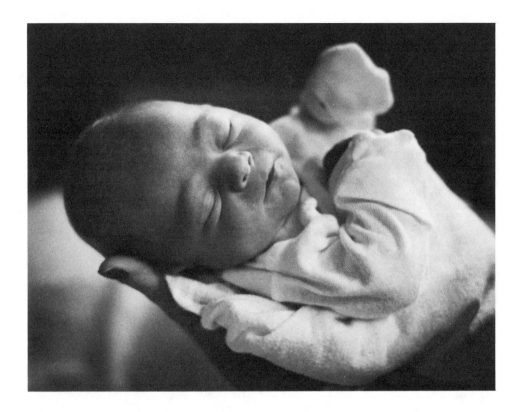

bed, trying to relax, count, and measure how far apart contractions were. When my husband arrived home at 11:00 p.m., the contractions were much stronger. Since we had quite a long drive to the hospital, he ran around the house getting my things together. I felt as if I were on the last dizzying slope of a roller coaster. I tried to keep track of the timing and found that adapted shallow chest-breathing helped. Although I felt a strong urge to tense my neck and shoulders and grip my hands, the breathing and focusing helped me maintain control. My husband brought me a wet washcloth to suck on, which also helped.

As we bundled ourselves into the van and headed for the hospital, the weather was far from favorable. There was ice on the road and snow swirled in front of us as we drove. I found a focus, kept up the breathing and began to feel a lot of pressure in my pelvis. The 45-minute journey seemed to take forever. My husband chatted away while I drifted in and out of the conversation, realizing that contractions were continuing to be about two minutes apart. What a relief it was to pull up to the hospital just before midnight and to be helped into a wheelchair. There was no way I could have walked! I was barely aware of being taken upstairs to the labor room. As I lay back on the bed, the nurse pulled off my boots and suggested that I take slower breaths, which helped. As my husband got scrubbed, the resident checked to see how far I was dilated. He was as surprised as any of us when he discovered that I was fully dilated! I had been in transition in the van!

Feeling a strong desire to push, I began pant-blow breathing. Two pants and one blow seemed to work best. On the way to the delivery room, the nurse helped me with my breathing, my husband stroked my arm, and they both encouraged me. "That's right. You're doing a good job."

In the delivery room I found another spot on which to focus and continued to pant-blow. The resident put my legs up into the rests, which were uncomfortably far apart until he adjusted them for me. Even though I was lying on my back, I was not at all uncomfortable. It felt good to have my legs supported and out of the way. I held the hand grips at the side of the bed when the doctor encouraged me to push, which was a great relief. My husband helped by counting loudly while I held each breath and pushed. Contractions were less frequent and I had time to relax more effectively between them. The atmosphere was casual and happy as people laughed and joked and talked about football!

Pushing felt good, but it was also painful. Somehow, I could concentrate on pushing better with my eyes closed, reminding myself of my Lamaze instructor's words, "Just remember, each contraction brings the baby's birth closer." I was aware of how close we were, and watched in the mirror as a small, hairy head became increasingly visible. The mirror was not all that easy to see, partly because it seemed so far across the room and partly because my doctor often positioned himself between me and the mirror, but the occasional view was enough to know what was happening. At last her head was out, and with the next push her shoulders and body followed. How exciting it was when the doctor held her up between my legs. Her eyes were wide open looking at me! "Welcome to the world, little one!" As she lay on my belly, I could feel her warmth, and my husband cut the cord with a flourish.

The placenta was easy to push out, and I was fascinated to see how thick it was. I was given a local anesthetic for the episiotomy repair. Since my legs and arms began to shake involuntarily, the nurses brought some hot towels for my chest and abdomen. The doctor massaged my tummy, which was quite painful as the uterus began to contract. Later in the recovery room the nurse did the same thing, but by then it was not so uncomfortable.

Melissa stayed with us for quite some time in the recovery room. She was hungry and nursed readily, remaining alert for about 45 minutes. How lucky I felt to have such a cooperative baby!

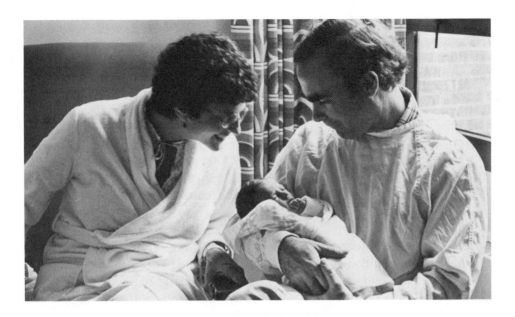

Richard is born

Our decision for this delivery was a birthing-room experience. My previous labors had been fairly short and easy, and the deliveries had progressed with no complications.

This was our third pregnancy. Each birth has been so different and exciting, although the pregnancies were similar—a weight gain of 25 pounds, swelling of lower extremities during the last weeks, leg cramps at night, and an occasional cervical cramping in the last month.

Nine days after my due date, I experienced mild lower-abdominal cramping similar to menstrual discomfort. These mild contractions were 15-20 minutes apart. Nine hours later they were five to seven minutes apart. After a half hour of contractions five minutes apart, we headed for the hospital. At this point I was having back discomfort, and my nerves were getting the best of me with uncontrollable shaking.

Our decision for this delivery was a birthing-room experience. My previous labors had been fairly short and easy, and the deliveries had progressed with no complications. At the hospital we were escorted to a birthing room of moderate size, complete with bathroom and shower. I was dilated to four centimeters. About two hours later my doctor arrived and ruptured the membranes to speed along labor. Within ten mintues I was in "first gear." Each contraction became harder and stronger and brought forth a gush of warm amniotic fluid.

By 4:30 a.m. contractions were two to three minutes apart. My husband combatted my lower-back discomfort by pushing my lower back as hard as he could with a cold washcloth and the heel of his hand. Although I was only five centimeters dilated, I felt as if I were experiencing transition. My lower extremities were cold and clammy. I was very restless, oblivious to what was happening elsewhere, and didn't feel like conversing. Lamaze breathing allowed me to remain in control, and the doctor suggested that I take a hot shower to help me relax.

How heavenly the hot shower felt as I sat on a stool in the shower. It warmed my cold skin and at the same time comforted my lower back. After two or three minutes, I experienced a hard contraction along with the urge for a bowel movement. Minutes later a very mild contraction occurred with no accompanying urge for a bowel movement. Minutes passed again until another hard contraction left no doubt in my mind— I wanted to push! I called for my husband. He pushed the panic button. I attempted some quick pant-blows, but the final stage happened with such speed that I panicked and bore down. My husband, doctor, and nurse were at my side in seconds. They helped me back to my bed which had been changed while I showered. A warming cart waited for the baby and lights remained low.

My next surprise was the doctor's decision to deliver this baby without an episiotomy if possible. My previous episiotomies had left quite a bit of scar tissue. I couldn't have been happier with his decision.

Pushing down seemed harder this time without a local anesthetic. I lay back in my bed, bending my knees, spreading out my legs, holding the head railings and my husband's hand. Instead of only three to four long, hard pushes (which I remembered from my previous deliveries), it took 15 minutes of pushing.

Richard made his appearance at 5:15 a.m. while my husband captured the entire birth with photos. Richard arrived wide-eyed and alert. He was wrapped in a warm receiving blanket and placed on my chest for us to touch and examine. My husband cut the umbilical cord, and the placenta was delivered within a few minutes. While the doctor examined the vagina for possible tears (I needed one stitch), my husband and I took turns holding Richard, and I took the very first father-son photo when Richard was fifteen minutes old.

After a while, the nurses put Richard in the warming cart and dropped silver nitrate into his eyes. Meanwhile an ice bag was applied between my legs to reduce swelling and ease the burning sensation of my vaginal area. The nurses checked my uterus and began kneading it to reduce the size. After 15 minutes or so, they were not pleased with how slowly the uterus was contracting. Blood clots began to accumulate, so I was given a synthetic hormone to promote contractions. It was injected into my buttocks, producing a very slight burning sensation for a few seconds.

Later I went to recovery instead of remaining in the birthing room. In recovery the nurse kneaded and pushed down hard on the uterus to eliminate the clots. My legs shook uncontrollably. A temporary catheter was inserted to rid my bladder of additional pressure. I learned later that my blood pressure had risen sharply and was closely watched until it dropped back to normal. This was a side effect of the synthetic hormone.

At 8:30 a.m. I went to my hospital room for breakfast, orientation, and our new baby boy.

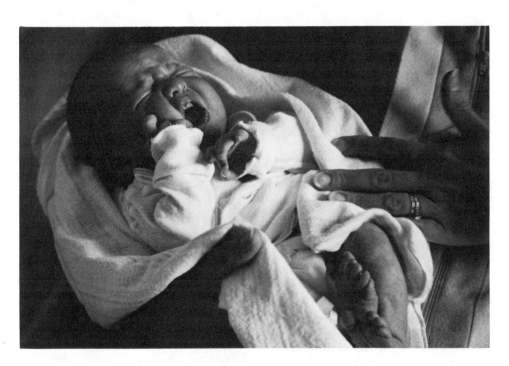

Kelly is born

The ambulance crew had been there only a minute when the baby's head was born. Since my husband and three of our four children arrived along with the ambulance, Kelly's birth on the family-room couch was truly a family affair.

Our little daughter entered the world in a rather exciting and unplanned manner. Around 2:00 p.m. Saturday afternoon, I began to feel an occasional tightening in the abdomen about every five minutes. Since I wasn't uncomfortable and it was still three weeks before my due date, I told my husband I was having Braxton-Hicks contractions or false labor and sent him out to do his errands in town.

At 2:30 p.m. I lay down to time the contractions, which were becoming stronger and more frequent, just to see if they were also **regular**. The contractions lasted about 30 seconds and came about every **two minutes. I used slow** chest-breathing, then switched to shallow chest-**breathing. Since the contractions** remained regular, at 3:00 p.m. I got up, closed my suitcase, changed my clothes, and lay on the family-room couch to wait for my husband.

At 3:30 p.m. I could feel the baby pushing down into the birth canal, so between contractions I undressed, put on my bathrobe, and asked my mother-in-law to call the ambulance and the hospital to let them know that today was "the day." I was using adapted shallow chest-breathing and then a light, shallow pant as I felt the bag of waters break. I continued to be very conscious of the step-by-step descent of the baby through the birth canal.

When the ambulance arrived at 3:38 p.m., I was concentrating on not pushing, in hope that I would make it to the hospital. At 3:40 p.m. when the ambulance crew had been there only a minute, the baby's head was born. As the ambulance driver unwrapped the cord from the baby's neck and suctioned mucus, her shoulders and body were born with a "swoosh"! Since my husband and three of our four children arrived along with the ambulance, Kelly's birth on the family-room couch was truly a family affair.

The ambulance driver wrapped Kelly and put her on my abdomen for the ten-minute ride to the hospital. There, a doctor cut the cord, and a few minutes later I expelled the placenta.

Unfortunately, our daughter developed aspiration pneumonia from breathing in amniotic fluid during her precipitous birth. Therefore, she remained in an isolette under 40 percent oxygen for a few days, where she was also warmed and treated for jaundice. We both went home when she was six days old, weighed six pounds, and was 19½ inches long.

After the birth, I didn't need any stitches and I felt wonderful. I am extremely grateful for my Lamaze training that allowed me to be in control of myself not only for my own sake but also for the sake of my family, who experienced a beautiful birth and saw me enjoying it too. My husband is also grateful for our Lamaze training, but he was disappointed that he missed the opportunity to participate fully.

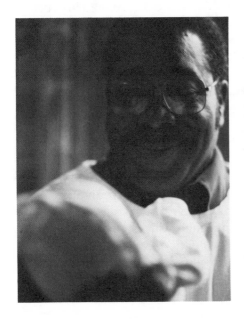
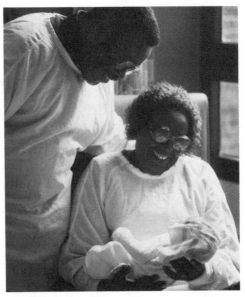

Brian is born

*Our obstetrician told us that babies are sometimes vaginally
delivered out of a frank breech position, but in our case she
inclined toward a cesarean delivery. This was my wife's first baby,
and given her age, 42, probably her only baby. She had also
already had four major pelvic operations. The doctor called this a
"premium pregnancy" and was determined not to take any chances.*

For months before our baby was due, it was clear that he was in the
frank breech position. You could easily feel the head doming up on the
left side of my wife's navel while the feet made visible lumps on the right
side and retracted if you tickled them. An x-ray made this graphically
clear: the baby was head up and very big looking, the little spine running
straight down like a railroad track, and the legs jack-knifed, bringing the
feet on a level with the head. Our obstetrician told us that babies are
sometimes vaginally delivered out of a frank breech position, but in our
case she inclined toward a cesarean delivery. This was my wife's first
baby, and given her age, 42, probably her only baby. She had also already
had four pelvic operations: one for appendicitis, two for ovarian cysts,
and one for a pelvic fracture. Since this baby meant a lot to us because

we wouldn't have another, our doctor called this a "premium pregnancy" and was determined not to take any chances.

It was possible, we knew, for babies to turn from breech position into the classical head-first approach to the birth canal. Our Lamaze instructor herself had had a breech baby who turned late in pregnancy. The possibility motivated us to keep doing the breathing exercises faithfully in preparation for a vaginal delivery, even though we didn't really think the birth would turn out that way.

A week after our last Lamaze class and a week before our estimated "B-Day," we toured the hospital. After the talk and tour, the nurse asked my wife if she was in labor and offered to check her out, but we were convinced that what she was having were Braxton-Hicks contractions. Unusually weary, we went home and climbed into bed at 9:30 p.m.

A little more than an hour later, my wife awoke with what felt like severe menstrual cramps. By the third one, she woke me. I ran and fetched a special bound notebook, and with an air of wild surmise, we began to time contractions and get through them with slow chest-breathing. With almost no variation, the contractions lasted 75 seconds and came every nine minutes. It was clear to us after a half hour that my wife was unmistakably in labor. For another hour and a half, we continued in fascinated devotion to the routine of counting and breathing, until the reality that "this was it" began to take hold and we recognized that something had to be done. So my wife went to the bathroom, we packed a little suitcase, and I called our obstetrician who, unfortunately, was out of town having board examinations. After reaching the doctor who was filling in for her (and who needed a little reminding—frank breech, first birth, 42 years old, previous pelvic surgery) we headed off for the hospital. All these interruptions definitely interfered with my breathing instructions and the clocking of the duration and interval of each contraction, but my wife continued the breathing patterns, which she found very useful.

"Hello again," said the resident as we walked into the delivery section. (He'd just seen us during the orientation tour.) From then on, a lot happened. The operation was set for 4:00 a.m. An intern came in and jabbed around, hunting for a vein for the intravenous feeding arrangement. The resident finally took over and found it. Off we went, the nurse and I wheeling my wife to x-ray to take another picture which turned out just like the one we'd seen before. By this time we were quite familiar with our baby's skeletal outlines. We saw his insides long before his outsides. After that, two anesthesiologists showed up to ask us what anesthetic we wanted. "Spinal," we said. The resident, a really pleasant person, appeared again with a paper to sign acknowledging that we understood that the operation entailed certain risks. Our doctor appeared calm, rough, kind, and possessed of that benevolence that comes from having faced a thousand crises and won. All the while, we were trying to count the duration and interval of the contractions, which were lasting about 60 seconds and coming less than five minutes apart. My wife was using shallow chest-breathing.

By dint of energetic insistence, our doctor had gained hospital approval for me to be in the operating room during the cesarean. As four o'clock approached, my wife was prepped and hauled off for the spinal anesthetic. I got scrubbed up, put on a sterile gown, a cap, socks, and a mask—and waited.

Meanwhile, in the operating room, the two anesthesiologists were having a go at administering the spinal block. They made four attempts, each one sending shooting pains down my wife's leg, but each time, blood appeared indicating a wrong placement. Finally the doctor decided to use a general anesthetic so there was no point in my being there during the operation. I waved to my wife, she waved back, and I left.

I leafed distractedly past one New Yorker cartoon after another in the fathers' waiting room, thinking about the inexactness of medical science and how one had to go ahead anyway.

In no time at all, the head nurse appeared. "You have a baby boy!" The next thing I knew, there he was—beautiful, rosy, squirming, rather groggy from the anesthetic, but certainly not in trouble for his life. "My wife's family nose," I thought. "My hair and mouth." In the recovery room, my wife, bandaged and festooned with tubes, asked over and over again, "Is it all right? What is it?" And I said, over and over again, "It's a beautiful little boy. Everything's fine."

It might look as if we didn't put our Lamaze instruction to much use. We only got into shallow chest-breathing and my wife was never dilated more than two centimeters. But we value the course very highly. Because of the classes and the close cooperation between our obstetrician, the hospital, and the Lamaze organization, we always felt we knew what to do, what the possible outcomes were, and what risks were involved. When things happened during the birth process and the time leading up to it, we knew what they meant. We had a map of the way, even though we had never travelled it before.

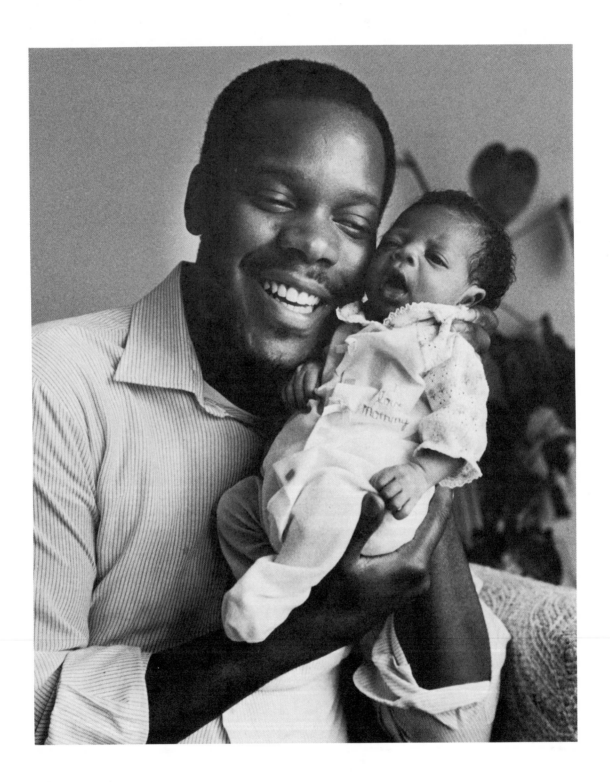

CHAPTER 7

Medical Assistance During Childbirth

Medical procedures

Induction—starting labor by artificial means—is attempted only when the baby is at term (fully grown), the woman's pelvis is big enough for the baby to fit through, and her cervix is soft and fully effaced. Attempts to induce labor without these prerequisites are usually unsuccessful. Health care providers undertake induction for medical reasons: diabetes, toxemia, Rh sensitization, premature rupture of the membranes without ensuing contractions, and a history of precipitous (very rapid) labor. Elective induction of labor may be a matter of convenience for the woman and her health care provider if she is at term but requires careful medical consideration. Labor is induced by the following methods, which may also be used in an attempt to enhance labor (make contractions more productive):

Induction of labor

- **Stripping of the membranes:** During a vaginal examination the health care provider gently separates the amniotic sac from the cervix without rupturing the membranes.

- **Rupturing the membranes (amniotomy):** During a vaginal examination the health care provider uses a sterile instrument, resembling a long crochet hook, to prick a small hole in the amniotic sac. The fluid released is generally clear, and you will feel the warmth of the amniotic fluid as it collects on an absorbent pad placed under your hips. After the procedure is completed, the amniotic fluid will continue to leak, necessitating frequent pad changes. Although the amniotic sac has no nerve endings, you may experience discomfort from the vaginal examination. After an amniotomy, your contractions may be closer together, longer lasting, and more intense.

- **Hormonal induction:** Oxytocin may be administered intravenously to stimulate contractions. After an IV is started, the amount of oxytocin given is increased until productive contractions occur. Hormonal induction is continually monitored by medical staff who also keep track of the baby, usually through the use of a fetal monitor.

Fetal monitoring   During normal labors, nurses periodically monitor mother and baby by feeling uterine contractions with their hands and listening to the fetal heart with a fetoscope or Doptone. When the medical staff feel the need to monitor and record uterine pressure and fetal heart rate continuously, they resort to electronic monitoring, which although continuous, does not alter or interfere with labor. Situations which call for electronic fetal monitoring through part or all of labor include vaginal birth after a cesarean, amniotic fluid stained by meconium (fetal excrement), premature labor, postmature labor, hormonal induction, prolonged labor, and the presence of maternal bleeding, twins, or fetal heart-tone inconsistency.

External monitoring, used in very early labor, involves two sensors which are secured to the mother's abdomen with an elastic belt. As the uterus contracts, the abdominal wall rises and presses against the first sensor. This sensor converts the uterine pressure into an electrical signal that is recorded on a graph. The fetal heart rate is recorded in a similar fashion by the second sensor. External monitoring is not very effective on obese women.

More accurate than external monitoring, internal monitoring is possible when the cervix is two to three centimeters dilated, the baby's presenting part is engaged in the pelvis, and the membranes have ruptured or can be ruptured safely. A small catheter is inserted through the cervix into the uterus to measure uterine pressure. A small wire is also attached to the baby's head. Uterine pressure and fetal heart rate are continuously recorded on a graph. Although the woman is confined to bed once internal monitoring begins, she may change positions as desired. The monitor can be detached for trips to the bathroom. Neither catheter insertion nor the monitoring process causes pain.

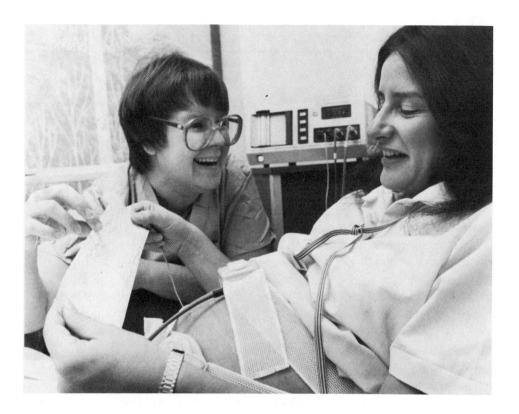

An IV may be started at any point during labor and usually is not removed until several hours after birth. The IV enables a woman to receive fluids, medication, or nutrition. Rapid breathing during labor and delivery gradually depletes the woman's store of water. If a woman cannot take fluids by mouth, hydration by IV is necessary. Additional fluid may also make it easier for her to urinate after delivery. An IV can rapidly introduce medication into a woman's system should an emergency arise. A woman may need an IV during prolonged labor in order to receive an energy-boosting glucose solution, or she may need an IV after delivery if she cannot take solids by mouth for several hours.

Intravenous fluids

Occasionally during labor, a woman does not feel her bladder filling with urine. Since a full or distended bladder takes longer to regain its tone, is easily infected, and may interfere with the baby's descent through the bony pelvis, catheterization may be in order. A nurse inserts a catheter into the woman's bladder, which drains the urine. Catheterization may also occur after birth, when tenderness and swelling of the perineum may

Urinary catheterization

interfere with the normal emptying of the bladder. If repeated catheterization is necessary, the catheter, emptying the urine into a drainage bag, may be left in for 24 hours.

Episiotomy

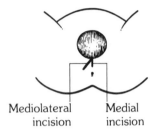

Mediolateral   Medial
incision   incision

During delivery as the baby's head comes through the birth canal, the muscular pelvic floor becomes thinner. Unfortunately, until the baby's head is born, it is difficult to tell whether or not the pelvic floor is thinning or stretching out sufficiently. Understretching may cause the pelvic tissues to tear, and overstretching may lead to a general weakening of the pelvic floor muscles. To avoid these problems and to ease delivery, the health care provider will probably perform an episiotomy, which is an incision in the pelvic floor muscles. The health care provider makes the incision, and following the delivery of the baby and the placenta, repairs the incision by stitching it with absorbable sutures. Although the local anesthetic will have numbed the area, it may not eliminate all sensation. If you are aware of some of the stitching, ask for more anesthetic, use slow chest-breathing, relax, and resist tightening the pelvic floor muscles.

Episiotomy discomfort is variable. Pain is caused as the tissues pull against the stitches. Resting quietly and applying ice during the first 24 hours reduces swelling and discomfort. You may also request a pain-relieving medication. After delivery a nurse will show you how to take a sitz bath, a basin of warm water in which you sit to relieve episiotomy discomfort and to promote its healing and cleansing. You may also apply medicated ointment to the sanitary pad to sooth the area of the incision and to prevent the pad from sticking.

Forceps delivery

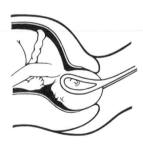

Forceps are used in the delivery room after the first stage of labor is completed. The physician may assist normal movement of the baby either by (1) rotating the baby's presenting part to a more advantageous position (from posterior to anterior position, for example) or by (2) providing downward traction to guide the baby through the birth canal. Forceps are hinged instruments of polished metal that look like large salad tongs and are shaped to support and guide the sides of the baby's head through the birth canal. Medical reasons calling for the use of forceps include fetal distress, a large baby, a woman who has had to push for a long time, or the use of an anesthetic which blocks the woman's urge to push.

Medications for labor and delivery

There are many medications available to help you relax and to relieve pain during labor and delivery. These medications are not intended to replace your own relaxation techniques and breathing patterns but may be used to supplement them.

Information about the common actions and side effects of available medications enables you to discuss medication with your health care provider during a prenatal visit. Knowing your medication preferences ahead of time allows your health care provider to consider your desires as medical decisions are made during labor and delivery. If medication is called for, understanding its action and side effects helps you and your partner to work with the medication, promoting maximum effectiveness. Remember, a Lamaze birth is a prepared birth, not necessarily one free from medication. Medication supplements Lamaze techniques. It does not replace them.

Your health care provider considers many variables before administering or withholding medications—your condition; the well-being, condition, and position of your baby; the course of your labor; and the duration and effectiveness of the medication. Preference for a particular type of anesthetic may also depend on the availability of a medical staff member proficient in its administration.

Throughout labor a nurse will monitor your pulse and blood pressure and your baby's heart rate. If you receive medication, the nurse will monitor you more frequently. She may start an IV, position you so that you are not lying on your back, or give you oxygen. She may give you medication to counteract side effects and reactions. She takes these precautionary measures to ensure the well-being of you and your baby.

There are four major types of medication that may be used during labor and delivery to aid relaxation or relieve pain—sedatives, tranquilizers, analgesics, and anesthetics. Sedatives produce a calming, quieting effect and, given in sufficient amounts, induce sleep. Tranquilizers help induce sleep, relieve tension and apprehension, and promote a state of calm and relaxation. Analgesics relieve pain without producing loss of consciousness. Anesthetics produce a loss of sensation and motor function with or without the loss of consciousness. Regional anesthesia provides pain relief to a specific region of the body while the person remains conscious. General anesthesia provides pain relief to the entire body by rendering the person unconscious.

Sedatives, tranquilizers, and analgesics

Medication	Action	Administration	Side effects on mother	Side effects on baby	Comments
Sedatives Barbiturates • Nembutal • Seconal	Promotes relaxation by reducing fear and apprehension. Induces sleep.	Time: Given in early labor, often when woman arrives at hospital and needs to rest before active labor begins. Method: By mouth, IV, or injection. Average duration: 4-6 hours with residual effects for up to 12 hours.	May cause excitement rather than relaxation.	Depresses baby's functioning. Baby may appear sleepy, limp, have poor suck, shallow respirations. Effects may last for several days.	Does not relieve pain.
Tranquilizer Phenothiazines • Phenergan • Thorazine	Reduces tension and apprehension. Reduces and helps control nausea and vomiting. Enhances action of narcotic analgesics. Phenergan has an antihistaminic effect. Thorazine is also an anticonvulsant.	Time: Given in early labor. Method: Intramuscular (IM) or IV. Average duration: 6-8 hours.	Dilates blood vessels. May cause drop in blood pressure. Drowsiness. Dizziness. Dry mouth.	Does not depress baby's functioning when used in recommended dosages.	Does not relieve pain.
Tranquilizer Benzodiazepams • Valium	Reduces anxiety. Induces sleep.	Time: Given after delivery. Method: IM or IV. Average duration: 6 hours.	Causes amnesia. If given in delivery room, mother will recall little of what happened there.	Produces a temporary lack of muscle tone.	Rarely given during labor because of depressive effect on baby. Given after delivery to help mother relax and sleep.
Analgesics Narcotics • Morphine Synthetic Narcotics • Demerol • Fentanyl	Reduces pain and tension without loss of consciousness.	Time: Given when labor is well established. Method: IM or IV. Average duration: IM—takes effect in 15-20 minutes and lasts for 3-4 hours. IV—takes effect in 15 minutes and lasts for 1-1½ hours.	Lethargy. Apathy. Dry mouth. Low blood pressure. Slowed breathing. Nausea.	Depresses breathing. Alters behavior if baby is born within 2-3 hours of administration.	May slow labor if given too early. When combined with Phenergan or Vistaril (a tranquilizer), action is enhanced and dosage can be reduced. Side effects are reversible when given with Naloxone (a narcotic antagonist).

Anesthetics

Name	Administration	Body parts anesthetized	Pros	Cons	Comments
Paracervical Block (regional)	Time: Given when cervix is dilated 4-7 cm. Method: Injected into both sides of cervix. Average duration: Immediate relief lasts 30-90 minutes.	Cervix. Uterus.	Does not affect the urge to push.	May give only partial relief.	Effect on baby is usually insignificant. 20 percent of babies do experience temporarily slowed heart rate (bradycardia).
Pudendal Block (regional)	Time: Given during second stage of labor (pushing and delivery). Method: Injected through vagina into tissue around pudendal nerve trunk located on each side of the pelvis at the level of the ischial bones. Average duration: 45-60 minutes.	Clitoris. Urethra. Vagina. Rectum. Perineum.	Safe for most women. Sufficient for large episiotomy repair and low forceps delivery. No side effects on baby unless baby is already in distress.	Woman may not feel actual birth sensation. May not be effective because of the difficulty of locating the pudendal nerve trunk.	
Epidural Block (regional)	Time: Given when cervix is dilated 4-7 cm. Method: Injected into back at waist level as woman sits or lies on side. Anesthetic goes into space that surrounds the spinal fluid sac. May be one injection or a continuous injection. Average duration: Takes effect within 30 minutes and continues through recovery.	Starts at waist and spreads down to toes depending on amount. Motor functions retained in rest of body.	Post-administration headache is less likely than with spinal or saddle block. Woman is conscious during delivery. No pain present during first, second, or third stages of labor.	May prolong second stage of labor by impairing urge to push and weakening abdominal muscles. May slow rotation of baby's head. May produce need for forceps delivery. May cause hypotension (low blood pressure). Requires large dose of anesthetic. Special skill necessary for administration. If dura (covering of spinal cord) is penetrated, entire spine may be anesthetized.	May be the anesthetic of choice for cesarean delivery. Electronic fetal monitor is necessary to monitor labor closely.

Anesthetics (cont.)

Name	Administration	Body parts anesthetized	Pros	Cons	Comments
Spinal Block and Saddle Block (regional)	Time: Given when delivery is imminent. Method: Injected into back at waist level as woman sits or lies on side. Anesthetic enters spinal fluid. Average duration: Takes effect immediately and lasts 1½-3 hours.	Waist to toes (spinal block). Perineum and inner thighs (saddle block). Feet can sense but not move.	Woman is awake for delivery. Requires low dose of anesthesia. Takes effect immediately. More predictable outcome than epidural block.	Blood pressure drops. Urination difficult. Urge to push is depressed. Low forceps may be necessary. Post-administration headache possible. May need to lie flat on back for 6-8 hours after administration. Entire spine may be anesthetized.	May be the anesthetic of choice for cesarean delivery or for prolonged second stage of labor.
Local Anesthetic	Time: Given immediately after crowning or after birth for comfort during episiotomy repair. Method: Injected into the perineum. Average duration: 30 minutes depending on type and amount.	Perineum.	Is safe for all women. Woman feels sensation of birth.		
General Anesthetic	Time: Given rarely for vaginal delivery unless problems preclude the use of regional anesthetics. For cesarean delivery, given after prep and draping. Method: Inhaled via mask, by IV, or through endotracheal tube. Average duration: For length of operation. Woman is drowsy for 2-3 hours after awaking.	Entire body.	Induces sleep-like state characterized by deep analgesia, amnesia, relaxation, and unconsciousness.	Woman unconscious for birth. Grogginess upon awaking. Sore throat. Vomiting and aspiration. Baby may be unresponsive or sleepy if analgesics are given prior to anesthesia or if delivery is delayed after administration.	For emergency or complicated vaginal delivery. For cesarean delivery.

Cesarean anesthesia

If you are anticipating a cesarean delivery, it is possible in some hospitals to make an appointment with the anesthesiologist prior to surgery to discuss your concerns and preferences. As they consider the anesthetic of choice for you, your physician and anesthesiologist look for the procedure that involves the minimum risk to you and your baby and provides relief from pain and discomfort.

There are a number of advantages to regional anesthesia. It provides effective pain relief, requires small doses of anesthetics, takes effect rapidly, and has little or no effect on the baby. In some hospitals, a spinal or epidural anesthetic to numb the lower half of the body is most frequently used for cesarean deliveries unless there are specific indications to the contrary. For the administration of a spinal or epidural anesthetic, the woman turns on her side with her legs flexed at the hips and knees. Her back at waist level is cleansed with an antiseptic solution and framed with sterile towels. First, the physician injects a small amount of local anesthetic to numb the spinal or epidural injection site. For a spinal block, the physician injects the spinal anesthetic into the sac of fluid that surrounds the spinal cord. For an epidural block, the physician injects the anesthetic into the space next to the sac of fluid that surrounds the spinal cord. This blocks nerves as they branch off the spinal cord. The level of anesthesia achieved in both cases usually extends from just below the woman's breastbone down to her toes.

Regional anesthesia

When a woman lies on her back following the administration of a regional anesthetic, she may experience sudden, severe nausea and vomiting. This results from the effects of the anesthetic and from lowered blood pressure. The pressure of the uterus on the veins which return blood from the lower extremities slows the return of blood to the heart, thus lowering blood pressure. To alleviate this problem, the woman can turn on her left side or hold her uterus on the left to relieve the pressure exerted by the uterus on the blood-returning veins. Hospital staff can administer oxygen, increase intravenous fluids, and give appropriate drugs to increase blood pressure.

With regional anesthesia, the woman is awake and can see and touch her baby right after birth, although she cannot see the operative procedure because a screen blocks her view. She may experience a strong pulling sensation in the lower chest and perhaps nausea just after the baby is delivered, but both sensations are short-lived. To promote complete relaxation and sleep after delivery, the physician may administer medication intravenously.

In most hospitals, a woman must be awake with spinal or epidural anesthesia in order for the father or partner to be present during a cesarean delivery. Thus, the woman who receives a regional anesthetic for cesarean delivery has the support of her partner and can enjoy her baby during those special first minutes of life.

General anesthesia For cesarean delivery, a general anesthetic is commonly used in cases of blood loss, severe toxemia, anesthetic sensitivity, fetal distress, or maternal preference. It is administered either by the inhalation of gases through a mask over the nose and mouth, by intravenous injection, or through a combination of these two methods. A tube is inserted into the woman's throat to provide an airway and to reduce her chances of aspirating stomach contents. In labor, intestinal motility and stomach emptying slow down, increasing the chances of vomiting and aspiration. Because of the airway tube, some women have a sore throat the day after general anesthesia. Because the medications used in general anesthesia cross the placenta from the mother's blood stream to the baby's, hospital staff closely monitor fetal heart tones as well as the mother's blood pressure, pulse, and respiration.

Birth experiences: Medically assisted childbirths

Following are actual birth experiences written by two women and one husband right after their children were born. Although these couples experienced a number of the procedures and medications described in this chapter, they also continued to use Lamaze techniques and to work together as members of a childbirth team.

Andrew is born

At 4:00 p.m. the doctor decided to discontinue the oxytocin drip so I could get some rest. By then I was exhausted, scared, and upset because everything seemed to be going wrong. I tried to sleep, but just as I was beginning to doze off, I began having strong contractions coming five minutes apart. I was in labor on my own!

On Thursday I awoke at 7:00 a.m. when the alarm clock went off. At first I thought maybe the baby had dropped during the night, causing my bladder to leak. Then I realized from the appearance of bloody show that my amniotic sac was leaking. Since I wasn't leaking badly or having any contractions, I decided to get some more sleep. About 7:30 a.m. my husband called the hospital, and they told us to come on in.

Looking back, I probably had some indication Wednesday night of the start of labor. I had been to see the doctor Wednesday morning. He did not do a vaginal exam. He said he'd see me next Wednesday and that I should expect the baby to be late. That night nerve pinches ran down my legs, which wasn't unusual, as I'd been getting nerve pinches throughout the last third of my pregnancy. They were, however, lasting longer and coming much more frequently than ever before. My husband thought they might be contractions and asked if he should time them. I said no, the baby was probably just dropping. I tried taking a hot shower but it didn't help. We went to sleep early and nothing else happened till Thursday morning.

By the time we'd dressed and arrived at the hospital, it was 8:30 a.m. I'd used three disposable diapers between 7:00 and 8:00 a.m.! As I still wasn't having contractions and felt fine, my husband parked the car in the parking lot, and we walked in together.

Since I'd been preadmitted several weeks earlier, we just reported to the admitting desk. They pulled my file and took us up to the examining room where I put on two hospital gowns. They examined me, decided that the amniotic sac really had ruptured, and found that I was only one centimeter dilated. My husband and I went to a labor room. At about 9:30 a.m., since I still wasn't having any contractions, my doctor ordered an IV with an oxytocin drip to try to induce labor. I was also hooked up to a monitor to record the fetal heartbeat and uterine contractions.

I began having contractions, but they weren't painful enough to use a breathing technique. In fact, I had to look at the monitor to tell when they were occurring. Throughout the morning and early afternoon, the amount of oxytocin was increased.

The nursing staff and doctors were terrific. They willingly showed my husband where he could find everything we'd need. They also phoned the nursing student who was following me through the pregnancy and post-partum period. She spent several hours with us in labor. At noon someone brought my husband a sack lunch. I was starving. All I'd had since Wednesday evening was a glass of juice.

About 3:30 p.m. the monitor quit, and at 4:00 p.m. the doctor decided to discontinue the oxytocin drip so I could get some rest. By then I was exhausted, scared, and upset because everything seemed to be going wrong. At 6:30 p.m. I finally had some dinner. My husband left shortly after 7:00 p.m. to go home, eat, and get some sleep. I tried to sleep, but just as I was beginning to doze off around 8:00 p.m., I began

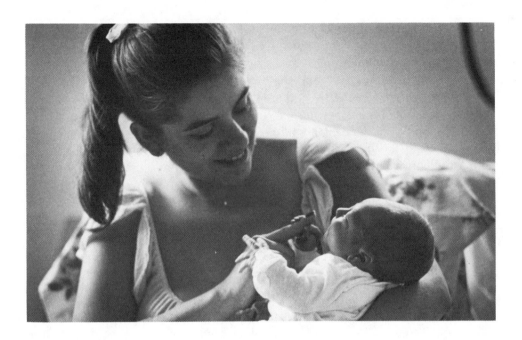

having strong contractions coming five minutes apart. I was in labor on my own! I called one of the nurses in. She stayed with me and helped me begin slow chest-breathing. When the doctor examined me at 8:30 p.m., I was four centimeters dilated. The contractions were coming closer together. Since I was having trouble controlling them, I switched to shallow chest-breathing and then adapted shallow chest-breathing.

When my husband arrived again at 9:30 p.m., I was nauseated and having a lot of difficulty controlling the contractions. I asked for a pain reliever and was given Demerol through the IV. Shortly after, I vomited. By about 10:30 p.m. I was eight centimeters dilated, which probably explains why I had difficulty controlling the contractions. Just before vomiting, I had been doing the pant-blow breathing with a lot of blowing, which made me hyperventilate, so I had to breathe into a paper bag. I was feeling the contractions as loin pains and did not realize I was in transition. The following is from my husband's point of view, as I lost all sense of time.

At this point, my wife devoted her entire concentration to keeping on top of her contractions, which were quite strong and long. After the Demerol she was able to maintain control fairly well, until about 11:15 p.m., when during a particularly intense contraction, she lost control. I pressed the call button long and hard, and half the staff poured in. She was nine centimeters plus, and soon reached ten. She was instructed to begin pushing, which she did with the nursing student and me assisting.

At about 11:40 p.m. my wife was moved to the delivery room. Transition had lasted about half an hour, and the birth itself took just half an hour. My wife achieved a relatively comfortable posture on the delivery table, was draped, and continued pushing with contractions. She didn't find much relief in pushing and had difficulty relaxing between contractions. The anesthesiologist gave her a pudendal block so she wouldn't feel the episiotomy, but it didn't detract from the actual sensations of the birth. The head emerged followed by the body shortly after. Andrew cried right after he was suctioned. He was placed on my wife's stomach while the umbilical cord was cut. He was born nine minutes past midnight, weighing six pounds, seven ounces. Here's my wife's point of view again.

Sewing up the episiotomy seemed to take forever. After the episiotomy was repaired, the doctor showed me the placenta, which I had asked to see. Andrew was brought to me in the recovery room for ten minutes, where I nursed him. At 2:00 a.m. I finally moved to my room. Both my husband and I were very excited. My IV was taken out at 6:00 a.m., and Andrew was brought to me for the 10:00 a.m. feeding Friday and stayed with me all day. He spent the first night in the nursery but was brought in for the 2:00 a.m. feeding and again for the 6:00 a.m. feeding, after which he stayed with me until I left the hospital.

I was glad I'd been able to see Andrew being born and to take care of him so soon after his birth. I had a bad head cold when I went into labor that made it difficult to use the breathing techniques we had practiced so faithfully.

The Lamaze preparation was great. The hospital staff was very supportive and knowledgeable about Lamaze and a big help when my husband wasn't there. They explained everything they did and answered all our questions. They said my husband was a big help to them in getting me to push as hard as possible. We will definitely use Lamaze techniques the next time around too.

Noah is born

Fred thinks the Demerol may have made me say some silly things, but it's difficult to know if I said them because of the Demerol or because of the back pain. Fred suggested constant back pressure, which really helped. I lay on my side and pushed back against his hand and was able to resist the urge to bear down.

We had many clues that labor was coming. The baby's head had been engaged for four-and-a-half weeks. I didn't experience a real burst of energy, but I was feeling much peppier and less lethargic than I had for a month. On Sunday morning I noticed a slightly pink-tinged mucous discharge and had one or two real contractions instead of the low pressure in the groin area that I had been having for several weeks. At 2:00 a.m. Monday morning, I was awakened by a hard contraction and quite a heavy, red bloody show. I timed the contractions at several intervals during the night, sleeping in between, and finally awoke Fred to help me time them at 4:30 a.m. They were very irregular, ranging between three and ten minutes apart and lasting from 30 seconds to 70 seconds. About 6:30 a.m. I passed a bright red clot, which seemed a little unusual to us. Since I had several contractions in a row at three-minute intervals, we decided to call the hospital to report the clot. They told us to come in. They checked to make sure that the red blood wasn't from the placenta. Since I was only a half-centimeter dilated, they sent us home with the reassuring advice that I'd probably have the baby within a week! The contractions stopped for the rest of the day Monday.

About 12:30 a.m. Tuesday, I woke up with a hard contraction and a slight gush of water. This was not an unusual nocturnal occurrence during the latter part of my pregnancy, but in the back of my mind was the idea that this might be my membranes rupturing, so I put on a sanitary pad and decided to stay up for a while to see what might happen. About 30 minutes later I began having hard contractions exactly five minutes apart, each with a small amount of fluid. With the fourth one of these contractions, my water really broke with a gush! I woke Fred as I rushed to the linen closet for a towel. After a call to the hospital we got ourselves together and arrived a little after 2:00 a.m. I wasn't at all effaced and still only a half-centimeter dilated.

The contractions stopped as soon as we arrived at the hospital. Since I hadn't slept much in the past 24 hours, they gave me morphine to make me sleep. Fred went to the fathers' room to sleep, and I dozed between contractions for about two hours. I was fairly comfortable on my side using the slow chest-breathing. Fred joined me at about 7:30 a.m. For the next five hours, the contractions were irregular, 20-60 seconds in duration, two to four minutes apart and there was bloody show with each contraction. I was comfortable using slow chest-breathing or often just effleurage.

At 11:00 a.m., the contractions stopped almost completely. Around noon the doctor decided to start an IV with glucose and water, as I hadn't had anything to eat since dinner Monday. They also decided to induce labor if nothing happened soon, since there was danger of infection if the baby wasn't born within 24 hours after the membranes ruptured. The pressure of the baby must have cut off sensation from my bladder, which the doctor discovered had become quite full on his examination at this point. Neither Fred nor I had realized that I hadn't had the urge to void at all. Partners should try to remind mothers about this.

About 1:30 p.m. they started the oxytocin through an IV, and I began having hard contractions one to three minutes apart lasting 40-60 seconds. Because someone had to monitor the contractions and fetal heart tones constantly (I understand this is always done when an oxytocic drug is administered), I found effleurage difficult—there wasn't enough room on my stomach for my hands along with the hands of everyone else! The slow chest-breathing kept me fairly comfortable. (I tried the

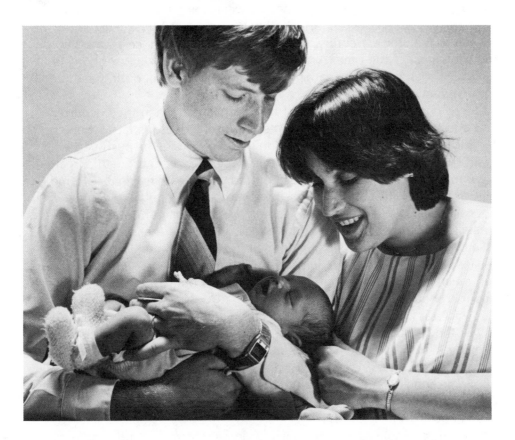

shallow chest-breathing and the adapted chest-breathing several times at this point and at the beginning of transition, but found them no more effective than the slow chest-breathing or, later, the pant-blow.)

From 2:00 to 3:00 p.m. I went from three to six centimeters and began having a strong urge to push. (I had wondered during Lamaze classes how I could recognize the urge to push, but there was no doubt when it happened!) I didn't see how I could pant-blow all the way to ten centimeters. This is when Fred proved an invaluable partner.

At about this time, the staff decided that the baby was posterior, which accounted for the severe back pain I was beginning to have. I was given Demerol which might have taken the edge off the contractions, but it certainly didn't make me feel light-headed the way the morphine had. Fred thinks the Demerol may have made me say some silly things, but it's difficult to know if I said them because of the Demerol or because of the back pain. Fred suggested constant back pressure, which really helped. I lay on my side and pushed back against his hand and was able to resist the urge to bear down. All the time, we were doing the pant-pant-blow breathing. This relief was short-lived, however, since it was difficult for the person to monitor my contractions with me on my side, so I ended up on my back most of the time. As a result, Fred had to work extra hard to make me stick with the breathing, and I did lose control during about half the contractions.

I recognized the symptoms of hyperventilation when they occurred, and you should have seen the expression on the doctor's face when, in the midst of complaining that I couldn't lay on my side or push yet, I quite lucidly told Fred to please get the paper bag we'd brought! Breathing into the bag helped me, but since Fred was breathing right with me, he was hyperventilating too. (I wish we had brought lip balm with us. The ice chips helped the inside of my mouth, but my lips got quite chapped.) I was also getting cramps in my upper legs. We found that when Fred did effleurage on them, it really helped me relax. After about 15 minutes, we realized that this was transition. The fact that we knew it wouldn't last too much longer was encouraging. As it turned out, transition lasted just about an hour.

At 4:15, I was dilated ten centimeters, and they told me I could push. It was the greatest feeling in the world! A nurse helped me by lifting my shoulders from one side and grasping my leg behind the knee to help me brace. I wish I'd had time to ask Fred to do the same thing. (He was lifting my shoulders from the other side.) I pushed about a dozen times in the labor room, during which the baby's head turned from posterior to normal position for delivery.

Fred got into a gown and mask while they took me to the delivery room. I was given a pudendal block, and because I was pretty tired by this time, the doctor decided to lift out the head with forceps. I pushed the head out half way and he finished with the forceps. In the delivery room I sometimes had trouble knowing when a contraction was over and when to stop pushing, but the nurse was a wonderful help by pacing the contractions for me with her hand on my stomach. The baby didn't cry till the doctor lifted him up for us to see that he was indeed a boy! I wasn't at all aware of the placenta being delivered, but Fred says it came almost immediately. I did experience some discomfort with the episiotomy repair because the pudendal block hadn't been completely effective and also because I had developed hemmorhoids while pushing, but we were so engrossed in our new son that this discomfort was of little consequence.

We just can't say enough for our Lamaze training. I did have a hard transition and wasn't able to control every contraction, but from our Lamaze sessions, we knew that transition wouldn't last too long. We were able to recognize what was happening at every step of the way, so even though my labor didn't follow the expected pattern, we were able to progress through it with confidence.

The most meaningful reward for me was having Fred with me. He had been somewhat unsure of his feelings about seeing the delivery, but after being with me all through labor, he was the most enthusiastic delivery room participant! I was very proud the next day when my doctor told me what a pleasure it had been for *him* to have Fred there, since Fred knew more about how to help me and make me comfortable than the doctor.

We were pleased, too, by the reaction of the medical students and interns who were with us during the labor and delivery. The medical students hadn't been on obstetrics long and hadn't had much experience with Lamaze-trained couples. They were very interested in the techniques and followed up by visiting me every day in the hospital to ask more questions! Needless to say, this did a great deal to add to our sense of accomplishment.

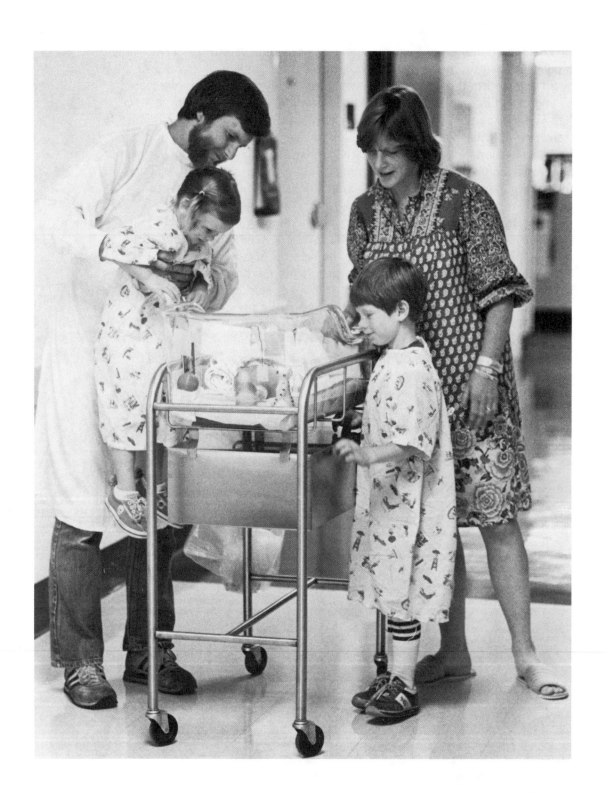

CHAPTER 8

After Your Baby Is Born

The mother's care in the recovery room

For one or two hours after you deliver, you will be observed in the room where you labored or in a recovery room. A nurse will frequently check your uterus, blood pressure, pulse, vaginal discharge, and episiotomy. Occasionally she may need to massage your abdomen over the top of the uterus with firm circular strokes until the uterus contracts effectively enough to prevent blood loss. The nurse will demonstrate this procedure so that you can check your uterus to see that it remains firmly contracted throughout the recovery period.

After a vaginal delivery

Often after delivery some parents relieve tension by laughing, crying, or talking excessively. These unexpected emotions can result from the physical and emotional exhaustion following labor and birth. To help you relax enough to rest and sleep, your partner can provide a soothing presence and even a backrub. You may have a light snack of fruit juice and toast.

For your comfort after delivery, your health care provider will probably order pain pills to relieve the discomfort associated with the early recovery period—the swelling of the vaginal area, the episiotomy, hemorrhoids, and the "after pains," or intermittent uterine contractions (rare after first deliveries but common after subsequent deliveries). If you are not in pain and do not feel you need pain medication, inform your nurse. Ice applied to your perineal area for the first four to six hours following birth will also help reduce the swelling and make you more comfortable.

If your bladder begins to fill in the recovery room, a nurse will give you a bedpan or help you to the bedside commode. Occasionally, because of swelling around the urethra or the effects of anesthesia, urination may be difficult and urinary catheterization may be necessary to empty your bladder.

After a cesarean delivery
Because a cesarean delivery is abdominal surgery as well as a birth, it requires a closely monitored recovery-room stay of two to three hours until your blood pressure, pulse, and respiration stabilize. Your feet may be elevated, and you may receive oxygen through a nasal tube. The nurse may massage your abdomen to promote effective uterine contractions. She will also check your abdominal dressing, monitor lochia, and inject pain medication for incisional pain. Your urinary catheter and your IV usually remain in place for at least 24 hours. If indicated, your physician may administer antibiotics orally or through your IV.

If you received a general anesthetic, the nurse will encourage you to cough and breathe deeply. As you do this, it is helpful to hold or splint your incision with your hands or a pillow. If you received a spinal or epidural anesthetic, the nurse will increase your activity level by having you bend your knees or raise your hips, although some anesthesiologists prefer that you lie on your back without raising your head for a period of time following spinal anesthesia.

Having a cesarean delivery does not prevent you from breast feeding or having your baby room-in. You can nurse your baby in the recovery room as long as both you and the baby are stable.

The daily routine during your hospital stay

When you leave the recovery room, you will go to your room in the hospital's postpartum unit where you will stay until you are discharged. The length of your hospital stay is an individual decision, but usually a woman stays for two to three days after a vaginal birth and for five to seven days after a cesarean birth. Although times and procedures vary from hospital to hospital, the following will give you a general idea of what to expect during a typical postpartum hospital day.

Your morning begins with the 5:00 a.m. feeding if your baby is staying in the nursery, or whenever your baby awakens if your baby is rooming-in. Your pediatrician or the pediatric nurse practitioner will pay an early morning visit to check your baby's weight, vital signs, and general well-being. Your health care provider will also check in with you to answer questions, discuss any concerns you may have, and see how you are adjusting to the new routines of postpartum life.

Morning (5:00 a.m. to 12:00 noon)

A nurse will take your temperature and pulse and check your episiotomy, after which you may wish to shower. For a few days you will probably perspire profusely, especially at night. This is one way your body eliminates the excess fluid you retained through your pregnancy and the fluids resulting from the reduction of uterine muscle tissue.

When your breakfast arrives, you may not have much of an appetite for the first day or two. After that you will probably be "famished" most of the time and will need to be careful to choose nourishing foods—extra fruit, milk, protein, and vegetables—rather than concentrated sweets. Your liquid requirements will continue to be about three quarts a day.

During the first morning you may still need an ice pack on your perineum to help reduce swelling around your episiotomy. After the first 24 hours, when the swelling is down you can begin taking sitz baths four times a day to promote episiotomy healing and comfort. For sitz baths, the hospital will give you a plastic basin that fits over the toilet seat. Fill the basin with warm water and sit on it for approximately 20 minutes. Taking a warm shower and letting the water flow over the episiotomy site is also soothing.

If you have had a cesarean delivery, a nurse will assist you the first time you sit up and the first time you walk. When you stand up for the first time, you may experience a "bearing down" sensation caused by the adhesive bandage around your abdominal incision. Don't be surprised or concerned if you also experience an increase in lochia when you first stand. Walking, deep breathing, and coughing (as you were shown in the recovery room) will hasten your recovery and help prevent complications.

After lunch, your afternoon will be taken up with napping, feeding, and caring for your baby; taking sitz baths; attending child care classes; and talking with friends and relatives who telephone or visit.

Afternoon (12:00 noon to 6:00 p.m.)

Relaxing and sleeping whenever possible is important. Mothers who do not rest enough usually become anxious and worry over minor occurrences. Postpartum "blues" are often precipitated by fatigue.

Many hospitals offer informal classes in general infant care, bathing, and feeding. Check with the nursing staff to see when classes are scheduled.

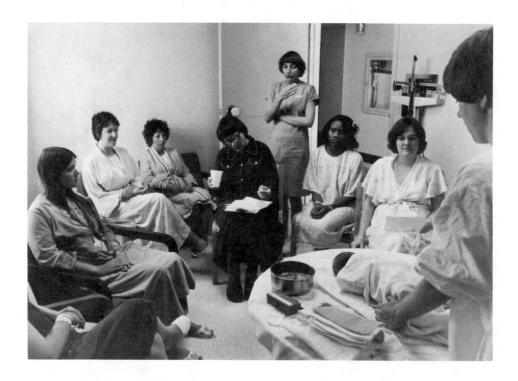

You will probably want to share this exciting time with relatives and friends. Remember, however, that visiting can be tiring. You may want to limit or space the number of visitors you have in the hospital and at home for the first few days or weeks.

Sometimes during the afternoon, a nursing mother should check her nipples for soreness or cracks. Ask the nurse for a breast cream which promotes healing. Also, try air-drying your breasts after each feeding. This helps prevent cracks and toughens the nipples.

Evening (6:00 p.m. to 10:00 p.m.) After dinner you may receive visitors, take another sitz bath, feed and care for your baby, have a snack, and retire for the night for some much-needed rest.

The nurse will encourage you to take a laxative before sleeping, since the first bowel movement after delivery can be uncomfortable. Increasing your fluid intake and eating fruits and roughage will also help.

Following a cesarean birth, some women find it difficult to urinate after catheter removal. If this happens, ask the nursing staff for suggestions. You will also be expected to have a bowel movement before you go home. Suppositories will help if you are having difficulty. If you experience discomfort from gas following a cesarean delivery, early ambulation, lying on your side or abdomen, or medication may help.

A snack will be provided for you during the evening. Be sure to select something, even if you are not hungry at the time, since you may be hungry later.

Feeding your baby: Getting started

Initially you will probably feel most comfortable wearing a supportive nursing bra for 24 hours a day. Absorbent nursing pads or clean handkerchiefs worn inside bra cups will help absorb leaking milk.

Breast feeding

Three to five days after giving birth, your breasts will begin to swell. This is called engorgement. It may last several days and is due to an

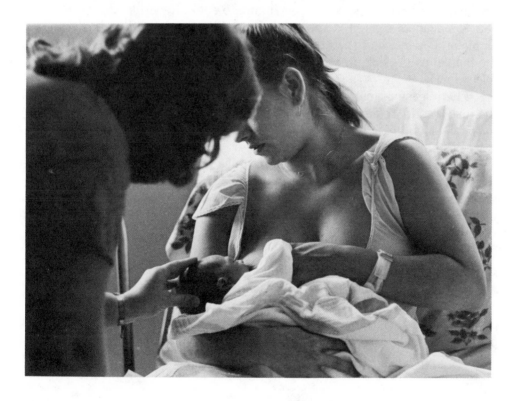

increased blood and milk supply in the breast tissues. Wearing a supportive, not-too-tight nursing bra, frequent nursing and hand expression of milk, taking warm showers, and putting a heating pad across your chest will ease engorgement discomfort and help prevent blocked milk ducts.

Some health care providers recommend nursing your baby on each breast for five to ten minutes each feeding the first day in order to prevent nipple soreness. If you do this, increase the baby's nursing time on each breast so that, by the third or fourth day, the baby is nursing on each breast for 15-20 minutes. Other health care providers believe that such careful timing is unnecessary and advocate, instead, letting the baby determine how long each nursing session should last.

Because the baby usually empties the first breast most thoroughly, you will want to alternate starting breasts so that, for one feeding, the baby starts on the left breast and, for the next feeding, on the right breast. To keep track of the starting breast, pin a safety pin to the bra strap of the breast the baby finishes with. This will remind you to start on that breast at the next feeding.

Many babies are somewhat sleepy after birth and may not be eager to nurse. Sometimes a baby may need to be encouraged to open his or her mouth to latch on to the nipple. A baby may like to lick the nipple at first and take some time before beginning to suck. Regardless of your baby's individual style, it is important for the baby to mouth both the nipple and as much of the areola (pigmented area of the breast around the nipple) as possible in order to stimulate the milk ducts in the areola to release milk.

The release of milk from the milk ducts is called the "let down" or the milk ejection reflex. You may experience this sensation in the hospital, or you may not become aware of it until you are home. Women have described it as a tingling sensation, a pins-and-needles feeling, or a sudden feeling of fullness in the breasts. Milk ejection will also occur in the breast not being nursed. You can press your forearm against this breast to stop the flow of milk. You may also experience this reflex when you hear your baby or someones else's baby cry, when you think about your baby, or after making love.

Bottle feeding Approximately six hours after birth, you or the nursery staff will give your baby a first feeding of water or sugar water. Subsequent feedings will consist of the formula prescribed by your pediatrician. Formulas are available in premixed, premeasured bottles or in concentrated liquid or powder that must be mixed with water. When you reconstitute concentrated liquid or powdered formula, be sure to measure the water and formula accurately.

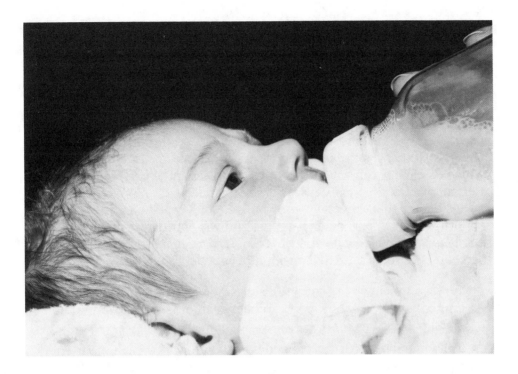

To give your baby a feeling of closeness and belonging, hold your baby during feedings. Babies whose bottles are propped up rather than held are apt to fall asleep with formula in their mouths, which can lead to tooth decay, ear infections, and choking.

If you have had a cesarean delivery, you may begin to breast feed or bottle feed your baby as soon as you feel able. Because of your incision, you may find it difficult to find a comfortable feeding position at first. You can use a pillow to cover and protect your incision. You can also ask the nursing staff for assistance.

Feeding after a cesarean delivery

Postpartum adjustments

The transition to parenthood is a time of particular stress when parents are especially vulnerable to the many changes occurring in their lives. Couples expect the feelings of love, joy, creativity, and closeness they experience with a new baby, but they may be unprepared for some of the negative feelings they are also likely to encounter. Your feelings and your mate's feelings about your new roles, shifting family expectations, hormonal and physical changes, marital adjustments, fatigue, household demands, your newborn's behavior, and anxiety about the challenges of caring for a new baby contribute to a period of disequilibrium for the entire family. These feelings may be especially strong after the birth of a first baby.

Individual reactions to both vaginal and cesarean birth are influenced by how each woman feels about herself; her expectations during pregnancy; the actual events of labor and delivery; and the reactions of medical staff, her family, and friends. For most parents, the birth of their baby is an exciting, happy time that may also be interspersed with times of disappointment, anger, depression, and inadequacy. When these feelings occur, share them with your mate, your health care provider, supportive friends, and other parents. You will find that many people have faced and coped with similar feelings. Here are some suggestions that may help you adjust to life with a new baby:

- With your spouse or partner, discuss how each of you shows and handles stress and how you can help each other during stressful situations.

- Talk together about the expectations you have for each other regarding feeding, bathing, and changing the baby and caring for older children; doing the laundry, preparing meals, and mixing formula; picking up toys; disciplining older children; arranging for babysitting; dealing with the needs and desires of grandparents.

- Read books, attend classes, and talk to other parents about parenting.

- Share your feelings about parenthood with your mate and other parents. Discuss with your mate what being a "good" mother or father means to you. Attend a mothers', fathers', or parents' discussion group if such groups are offered in your area.

- Together with your mate, plan ways you can both get plenty of rest and sleep, especially in the early weeks.

- Enlist the help of relatives and friends. They can help with household chores and child care. Public health nurses will also help you as you learn to care for your newborn baby.

- Plan ahead for child care if returning to work or school. Find out about the place and people who will be caring for your baby, and gather references from other parents.

- If one parent is working and the other is staying home with the baby, discuss ways you can both make time for intellectual, social, and creative stimulation.

- Talk about how the baby will affect your social patterns, vacation habits, or travel plans.
- Discuss financial priorities, especially if one parent has stopped working to care for the baby.
- Talk with your mate about your feelings about sex. Most parents find that having a baby changes their sex lives somewhat.
- Give yourself time. Remember, as parents you are more than caretakers of a baby. You are partners in a unique relationship that needs time to develop and grow.

Postpartum exercises

These exercises will help restore muscle tone after your baby is born. You may start some of these exercises while you are still in the hospital. Check with your health care provider, however, before beginning any exercise program.

This exercise teaches you to relax the pelvic floor muscles, which help prevent involuntary urine leakage. It also strengthens the muscles that support the bladder, urethra, vagina, uterus, and rectum. To begin, slowly tighten the urethra as if to stop the flow of urine. Next, tighten the muscles that surround the vagina and feel your pelvic floor lift. Finally, tighten the sphincter muscle around the anus. Hold for five seconds, and slowly release. Next, lie on your back on the floor with your legs extended and your head on a pillow. Tighten the muscles that surround the urethra, the vagina, and the anus, and without tensing your abdomen or thighs, cross and uncross your ankles. Release your pelvic floor muscles from front to back and repeat the entire exercise.

Advanced Kegel exercise

This exercise promotes lower-back muscle flexibility. (See instructions in Chapter 3.)

Back stretching

This exercise is good for your thighs and lower-back muscles. Lie on the floor on your back with your legs extended straight out on the floor, your pelvis tilted, and a pillow under your shoulders. Keeping your left leg straight, bend your right leg by sliding your right heel back along the floor, in toward your buttocks as far as it will go. Then slide your right

Leg sliding

heel forward to resume an extended right leg position. Repeat with the left heel, keeping the right leg straight. When you are able, do this exercise working both legs simultaneously but in opposite directions—as you slide your right heel forward, slide your left heel backward.

Leg sliding

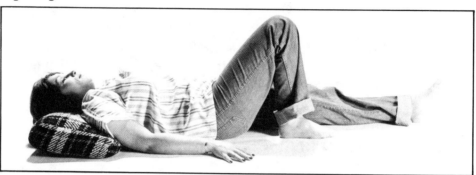

Leg bicycling This exercise stengthens your inner thigh muscles and stretches your calf muscles. Lie on your back with your legs straight up in the air, toes pointed, arms at your sides, palms on the floor. Draw your knees to your chest. Extend the right leg keeping the left knee bent to your chest, then extend the left leg drawing the right knee to your chest. Repeat this motion as if you were riding a bicycle.

Thigh lifts This exercise stengthens your outer thighs. Lie on your right side with legs extended, toes pointed, right arm extended straight out on the floor above your head and the left arm bent so that the palm is pressed into the floor at your bustline. Slowly raise your left leg to the count of eight and slowly lower it to the count of eight. Roll over to the left side and repeat with the right leg.

Leg bicycling

Thigh lifts

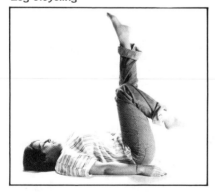
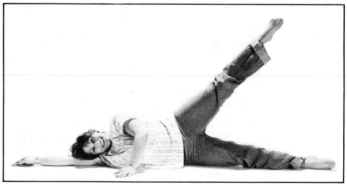

This exercise will help reduce your waistline and strengthen your waist **Waist stretch** and back muscles. Stand with your feet about 12 inches apart and stretch your arms above your head. Slowly bend at the waist from side to side stretching as far as possible. Bend directly to the side keeping your shoulders in line with your hips.

These exercises restore your abdominal muscles, especially after a **Abdominal** cesarean delivery. (1) Lie on your back with your knees bent and your **tightening** feet flat on the floor. Take a deep breath through your nose, keeping your ribs as still as possible and letting your abdomen expand upward. Part your lips slightly as if blowing out a candle, and blow out slowly and forcibly, pulling the abdominal muscles in until you cannot blow anymore. Repeat in sitting and standing positions. (2) Lie on your back with your knees bent and your feet flat on the floor. Curl your head and shoulders off the floor as if you were trying to look over your abdomen. Feel the tension in your upper abdominal muscles. Lower your head and shoulders slowly to the floor.

Waist stretching

Abdominal tightening

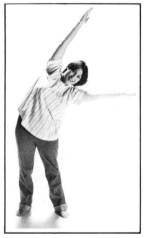
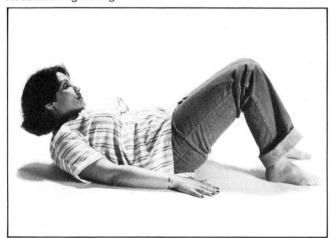

This exercise increases the strength and tone of your lower abdominal **Pelvic tilt** muscles, increases the flexibility of your back, promotes good pelvic alignment, relieves pelvic congestion, and helps prevent and relieve lower backache. (See instructions in Chapter 3.)

This is good for your back and abdominal muscles. Sit on the floor with **Curl downs** your knees bent, feet flat on the floor, hands on knees, pelvis tilted, back rounded, and abdominal muscles tightened. From this position, gradually lie back as far as you can while maintaining a curved back and pelvic tilt. Return to a sitting position and repeat.

Curl downs

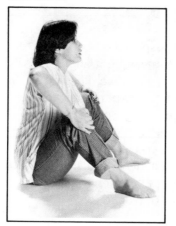 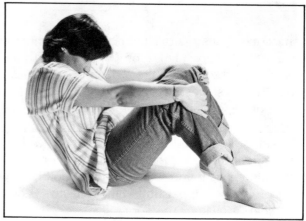

Contraception

Health care providers have differing opinions about when couples can resume sexual intercourse after childbirth. Occasionally abdominal or pelvic floor healing can delay the resumption of intercourse. If you are breast feeding, vaginal secretions will be decreased and intercourse may be uncomfortable, but you can alleviate this problem by using a lubricating preparation. If you are uncertain or uneasy about resuming intercourse, discuss your feelings and concerns with your health care provider and your mate.

Resuming sexual intercourse after childbirth can be like "starting all over again." For some couples this is an exciting, rewarding experience, while for others it is a time of confusion and uncertainty. Remember to express your feelings to one another in either situation and give yourselves plenty of time, support, and encouragement.

The following charts describe various methods of birth control. Not all methods are suitable immediately after childbirth, however, so you may have to choose a temporarily less satisfactory method until your body returns to its pre-pregnant state. If you are breast feeding, do not rely on breast feeding as an effective means of contraception, and do not plan to use oral contraceptives until after your baby is weaned. If you have questions and concerns about postpartum contraception, discuss them with your health care provider or pharmacist.

Methods of contraception

Name	Description	Effectiveness	Possible side effects	Cost	Pros	Cons
Oral Contraceptives (The Pill)	Beginning on the fifth day of her menstrual cycle, a woman takes 1 pill each day for 21 days, stops taking the pill for the next 7 days while she menstruates, and begins the 21-day cycle again. (The number of days in the cycle varies depending on the pill prescribed.) Hormones in the pills inhibit ovulation and produce a change in the lining of the uterus.	Is the most effective birth control method except for sterilization. When pills are taken regularly, only 0.7-1.4 women per hundred women become pregnant over the course of a year.	Weight gain Nausea Breast tenderness Increased or decreased sexual drive Abnormal blood clotting Decreased menstrual flow	$7-$10 a month (less from a family planning clinic)	Is extremely reliable. Permits spontaneous intercourse without preliminary preparations. Regulates menstrual periods. Lightens menstrual flow.	Produces side effects. Cannot be used while breast feeding. Must be prescribed by a physician who knows woman's medical history.
Intrauterine Device (IUD)	A copper, plastic, or stainless steel device is inserted into the woman's uterus. It is thought to work either by causing a mild inflammation in the uterine lining, which prevents implantation of the fertilized egg; by causing a chemical change in the uterine fluid, which destroys the sperm; or by moving the egg through the tube rapidly enough to prevent implantation.	Is second only to "the pill" in effectiveness. Results in 2-4 pregnancies per 100 women per year.	Cramps Heavy menstrual flow Irregular bleeding and expulsion Pelvic infection Uterine infection If pregnancy does occur, an increased chance of ectopic pregnancy (gestation outside the uterus, often in a Fallopian tube) or miscarriage	$30-$50 for insertion (less from a family planning clinic)	Is reliable. Permits spontaneous intercourse without preliminary preparations. Side effects are rare.	Produces side effects. Must be inserted by a physician who knows woman's medical history.
Condom (Rubber)	A thin sheath of rubber, latex, or animal membrane is placed over the man's erect penis to prevent sperm from entering the woman's vagina during intercourse.	Used correctly and consistently in combination with contraceptive foam, results in probably less than 3 pregnancies per 100 women per year.	Allergic reaction to rubber, latex, or animal membrane (rare)	$.35-$1.25 each (less from a family planning clinic)	Provides protection from venereal disease. Is available without prescription. Is used only during intercourse.	Interrupts intercourse. Decreases physical sensitivity. May be uncomfortable after childbirth unless used with lubrication.
Rhythm Method	Most women ovulate (release an egg from the ovary) once a month. If a woman can determine when she ovulates, by taking her temperature each morning, she abstains from intercourse during this period. This method should be supervised by a physician.	Because of irregular menstrual cycles and long periods of abstinence, the pregnancy rate is 14-40 per 100 women per year.	Fear of pregnancy Pregnancy	$5 for a basal temperature thermometer	Uses no chemicals. Is sanctioned by the Roman Catholic Church.	Exact time of ovulation is difficult to determine. Some women ovulate more than once a month. Long periods of abstinence from intercourse required during the ovulatory period.

Methods of contraception (cont.)

Name	Description	Effectiveness	Possible side effects	Cost	Pros	Cons
Diaphragm	A soft rubber or latex dome with a flexible metal rim, used in combination with spermicidal cream or jelly, is placed over the woman's cervix to prevent sperm from entering the uterus during intercourse.	Used correctly and consistently, results in about 3-5 pregnancies per 100 women per year.	Allergic reaction to rubber, latex, or spermicide (rare) Increase in urinary tract infections	$10-$12 plus physician's fee for fitting (less from a family planning clinic)	When fitted correctly and inserted properly, is not felt by either partner. Can be inserted 4 to 6 hours before inter-·course.	May be difficult to insert. Insertion at time of intercourse may interrupt spontaneity. Can be improperly inserted. Must be left in place 6 to 8 hours after intercourse. Must be checked frequently for holes. Must be checked yearly for size by physician.
Cervical Cap	Looks like a large rubber thimble with a thick rim. It fits snugly over the woman's cervix and is held in place by suction. Prevents pregnancy by blocking sperm at the entrance of the uterus. Is used with a spermicide.	Is as effective as a diaphragm.	Allergic reaction to rubber or spermicide (rare) Effects of continuous suction on cervical tissue (under investigation)	Currently an experimental device. May be obtained by women who volunteer to participate in an FDA-approved study. Initial cost $45-$55. Follow-up visits $10/visit.	Is convenient. May be left in place for up to 3 days. Permits spontaneous intercourse. Is safe. Has no effect on future fertility.	Causes occasional discomfort from feeling the cap. May cause cervical irritation (rare).
Chemical Vaginal Contraceptives	Foam placed deep in the vagina forms a spermicidal barrier over the cervix. Creams, jellies, and suppositories inserted into the vagina kill sperm on contact.	Foam used alone permits about 18 pregnancies per 100 women per year. Used in combination with a condom, permits about 3 pregnancies per 100 women per year. Creams, jellies, and suppositories are better than no protection at all, but are not highly reliable.	Allergic reaction to foam, cream, jelly, or suppository A heat-related reaction, irritating to woman and partner, with some suppositories	$6 for foam kit with applicator. Creams, jellies, and suppositories cost less (available from a family planning clinic).	Is available without prescription. Is used only during intercourse. Is inexpensive.	May cause irritation. Must be inserted only a few minutes before intercourse. Insertion may interrupt intercourse. Is not highly reliable.

Methods of contraception (cont.)

Name	Description	Effectiveness	Possible side effects	Cost	Pros	Cons
Billings Method	This natural method requires abstinence from intercourse for a 7- to 9-day period surrounding ovulation. In each cycle a woman can predict the approach of ovulation by a discharge of sticky mucus at the vaginal outlet several days before ovulation. Right around ovulation, the mucus becomes less tacky. Post-ovulatory days usually feel "dry" to the woman. In some cases, a basal temperature thermometer may be used. Method taught at clinics and in special classes.	Fewer than 4 pregnancies per 100 women per year claimed. Method too new for reliable statistics, however. Effectiveness increases when combined with rhythm method.	None	None unless a basal thermometer is purchased	Uses no chemicals.	Requires abstinence from intercourse during the ovulatory period.
Male Sterilization (Vasectomy)	In this simple, outpatient surgical procedure a section of the vas deferens (the duct which carries sperm to the ejaculatory duct) is removed, rendering a male permanently sterile.	Is at least 99% effective. However, another contraceptive method is necessary until the male reproductive system is cleared of residual sperm.	Swelling, tenderness, or infection following surgery	$135-$175	When proper precautions such as follow-up semen analysis are done, should be 100% effective in preventing pregnancy. Some couples report ehanced sexual enjoyment because they no longer fear pregnancy.	At present, sterilization should be considered irreversible. A couple should consider the possibility of the death of existing children or the death of a partner, divorce, and remarriage. They should be certain that their family is complete before undergoing sterilization.
Female Sterilization (Tubal Ligation or Laparoscopy)	In this surgical procedure an abdominal incision is made and a section of each Fallopian tube is removed and tied or cauterized, preventing eggs or sperm from passing through the Fallopian tubes.	Considered 100% effective and permanent.	Risk of surgical and anesthetic complications Postoperative discomfort	$250 if done immediately after childbirth. More if done later due to additional hospitalization costs.	Without the fear of pregnancy, sexual relations may be more relaxed and enjoyable. In some cases, Fallopian tubes can be surgically rejoined.	(Same as for male sterilization).

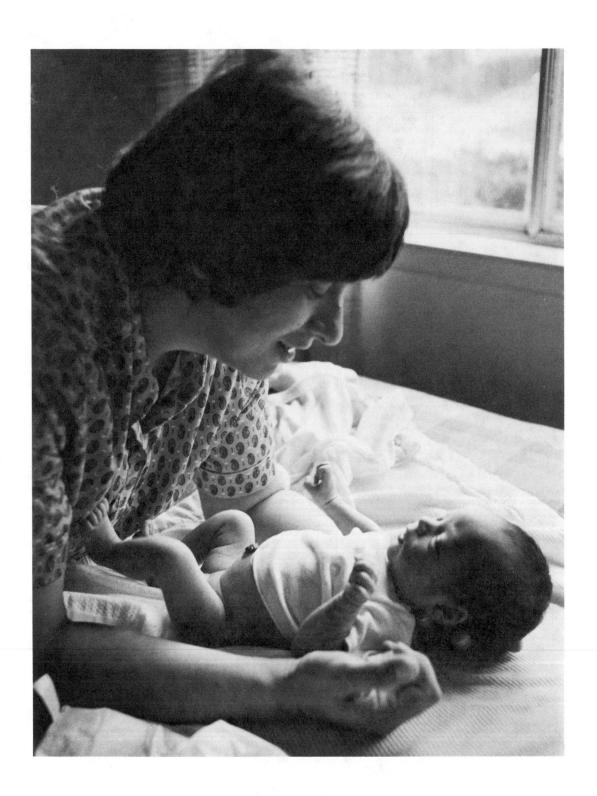

CHAPTER 9

Your Newborn Baby

Bonding

Bonding is a complex set of responses and behaviors involving parents and their offspring. These responses and behaviors ensure the survival of the species when the offspring are helpless and vulnerable. Human babies need daily care, protection, and nurturing by their parents, at first to survive and later to develop and learn. Babies usually bond or become attached to their parents or parent surrogates through close, consistent contact. While some parents imagine that bonding is an instant, automatic instinct permanently joining them to their baby the minute after birth, this is not so. Bonding or attachment is a gradual process that actually begins in utero and continues after birth as parents and babies meet, touch, and communicate.

New babies and parents are physiologically primed to respond to each other. In fact, right after birth, many babies have a quiet, alert time when they are particularly responsive to cuddling, fondling, being talked to, feeding. This initial contact between baby and parents is the beginning of a life-long relationship.

Sometimes circumstances prevent parents from spending time immediately after birth with their baby. The mother or baby may need immediate medical attention, for example. Even though priority medical procedures may interrupt the bonding process, the mother's and father's support and love remain essential to their baby's physical and emotional development. When a baby is born prematurely or when the baby or

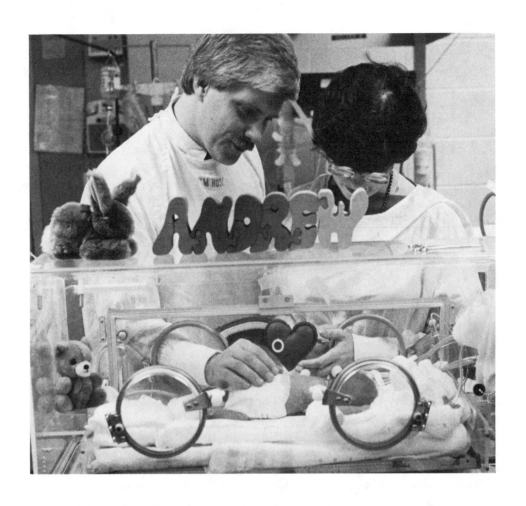

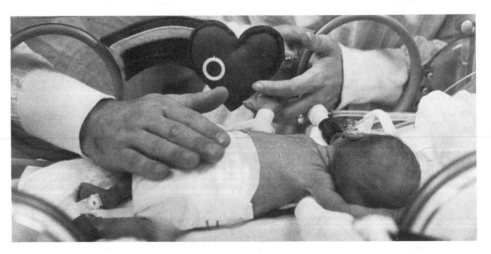

mother is stressed, traumatized, or ill, the family's bonding and attachment process can continue with some modifications.

Parents of a premature baby who requires immediate intensive care in a specially equipped nursery are extremely vulnerable to a number of feelings and emotions. They may feel guilty and responsible for everything that happens to their baby. They may grieve over the loss of the "perfect" baby they had anticipated and over the "defects" in the baby they produced. They may blame themselves for the baby's condition. It is much easier, however, for parents of hospitalized premature babies to come to terms with their feelings when they are allowed to participate in the baby's care in the high-risk nursery. There they can touch and talk to their baby, work out their anxieties, and get to know their baby before they take the baby home. Hospital staff in intensive-care nurseries usually go out of their way to help parents adjust to their baby's condition and to include parents in the baby's care.

Newborn characteristics

To most parents their newborn baby is beautiful. Far from it! For one thing, newborn babies are usually covered with vernix caseosa (the cheese-like covering that protected the baby in the uterus). This will eventually wear off on its own. If it persists in the creases and folds of the skin, however, you can gently wash it out with soap and water. In general, a newborn baby's skin is wrinkled, creased, and blotchy for the first few weeks or so. Patches of pimples will come and go. A baby whose delivery was assisted by forceps may have red marks on the cheeks where tiny blood vessels ruptured. As the blood vessels repair themselves, these marks will fade and disappear. A baby may have red birthmarks on the bridge of the nose, on the eyelids, or on the nape of the neck. These, too, will fade with time and the one on the neck will be hidden by hair. After a few days, a strawberry birthmark may appear anywhere on the baby's body but usually on the chest or face. This red, raised patch gradually fades and often by the age of three will be gone altogether.

Around the second or third day, your baby's skin may turn yellowish. This is physiological jaundice, which occurs when excess red blood cells break down into bilirubin. In most cases, physiological jaundice disappears on its own. If blood tests indicate high levels of bilirubin, however, the pediatrician may place your baby under lights to promote the elimination of bilirubin. This may result in a longer hospital stay for

Appearance

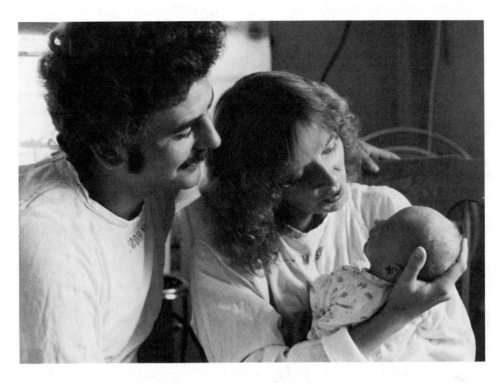

the baby. If high bilirubin levels are not treated, however, they may lead to problems in the baby's development.

Some babies are born with quite a head of hair. Others enter the world almost completely bald. In either case, new hair will begin to grow when the baby is about six months old. With or without hair, however, a newborn baby appears to have a large head, because at birth a baby's head is one third of adult size while its body is only one twentieth of adult size. On top of the baby's head is a soft spot where four bones of the skull have not yet grown together. These bones will join when the baby is about 18 months old. In the meantime, the soft spot, or fontanelle, is covered with a tough membrane so that the baby is not too vulnerable at that spot.

Because the baby's fingernails and toenails grow in the uterus, soon after birth they may need cutting with a fine pair of scissors for the baby's own protection.

The baby's breasts may swell for a few days in reaction to the same hormones that stimulate your milk production. This swelling will disappear on its own.

It may take two to three weeks for your baby's umbilical cord to shrivel, turn brown, harden, and fall off. Your pediatrician will give you specific cord-care instructions. In general, however, keep the following suggestions in mind:

- Keep the cord as dry as possible.
- Fold the diaper below the cord.
- If the cord sticks to the baby's shirt, remove the shirt gently.
- Do not totally immerse your baby in the bath until the cord detaches.
- If there are flecks of blood at the base of the cord, wipe with an alcohol swab three or four times a day.
- Greenish discharge, foul smell, or redness may indicate infection. Contact your pediatrician.

If your baby boy has been circumcised, the incision will probably heal on its own. Wash the incision with clean water each time you change his diaper. If the penis has been wrapped in gauze, remove the gauze when it begins to get soiled. Do not rewrap. A few drops of blood are normal. If you notice any of the following signs of infection, however, report them to your pediatrician: redness, pus-filled drainage, tenderness after the third day, blood-streaked urine, reduced urination (dry diaper after eight hours).

Vision

From birth, your baby is able to see, respond to human faces, focus on patterns with bright colors and on shiny objects that reflect light, and shut the eyes against bright light. Your baby will enjoy eye-to-eye contact with you especially when you also touch, stroke, murmur, talk softly, smile, and kiss your baby. Your baby will let you know that he or she enjoys your attentions by mirroring your facial expressions, sticking out or clicking the tongue, sucking, and vocalizing. Your baby's clever antics will delight you, and your baby will enjoy your attention.

Bowel habits

Each baby has unique bowel habits. Your baby's bowel movements may come many times a day or every few hours. The first bowel movement, called meconium, is dark and sticky. Gradually the bowel movements of breast fed babies become frequent, loose, and yellow; bottle fed babies have bowel movements that are yellow and more formed. If bowel movements are hard and dry, your baby may be constipated. A frequent wet diaper, on the other hand, means that your baby is getting enough fluid.

Sleeping and waking

Many babies spend their first few days of life sleeping. Some babies wake up only for feedings and then drop right back to sleep. For the first few days, they often sleep in the same position they assumed in the uterus. Gradually, however, they will sleep in more comfortable-looking positions and will spend more and more time awake.

Babies have various levels of sleep and wakefulness. A baby in a deep sleep will resist attempts to be wakened and fed. On the other hand, a baby in light sleep might either be aroused and fed easily or slide into a deep sleep and resist arousal. Since a baby's behavior in each level of sleeping and waking is fairly consistent, you can predict your baby's reaction to feeding, bathing, diaper-changing, cuddling, playing, or talking, depending on your baby's sleepiness or wakefulness.*

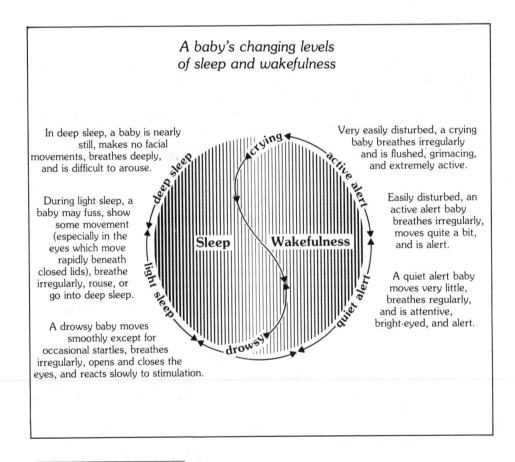

A baby's changing levels of sleep and wakefulness

In deep sleep, a baby is nearly still, makes no facial movements, breathes deeply, and is difficult to arouse.

During light sleep, a baby may fuss, show some movement (especially in the eyes which move rapidly beneath closed lids), breathe irregularly, rouse, or go into deep sleep.

A drowsy baby moves smoothly except for occasional startles, breathes irregularly, opens and closes the eyes, and reacts slowly to stimulation.

Very easily disturbed, a crying baby breathes irregularly and is flushed, grimacing, and extremely active.

Easily disturbed, an active alert baby breathes irregularly, moves quite a bit, and is alert.

A quiet alert baby moves very little, breathes regularly, and is attentive, bright-eyed, and alert.

deep sleep · crying · active alert · Sleep · Wakefulness · light sleep · drowsy · quiet alert

*For further information about sleep and awake states, see *Neonatal Behavior Assessment Scale* by T. Berry Brazelton.

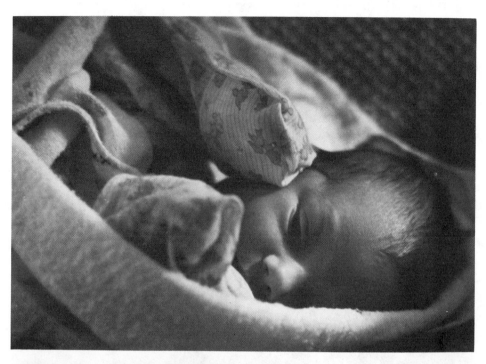

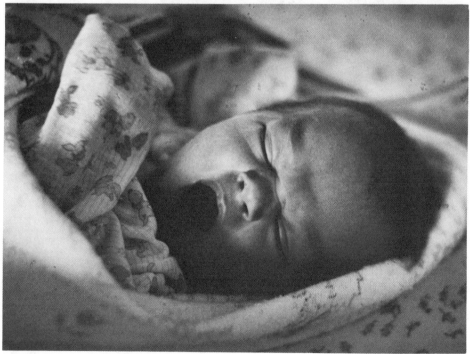

Reflexes, signals, and cues

Reflexes Because they are so small, newborn babies may look more helpless than they actually are. At birth, however, they already possess many abilities. You can appreciate these abilities by looking for your baby's reflexes— predictable behaviors normally present at birth. For example, your baby's head will automatically turn toward the right when you stroke the baby's right cheek and toward the left when you stroke the left cheek. This "rooting" reflex helps your baby find your nipple for nursing. At first, a nursing mother and baby will be unaccustomed to the movements and sequence of searching, rooting, and finding the nipple. Most babies, however, will repeat their successes and soon learn where the milk is.

Grasping is another newborn reflex. When you place your finger in your baby's grasping hand, the grasp is so strong you can pull your baby

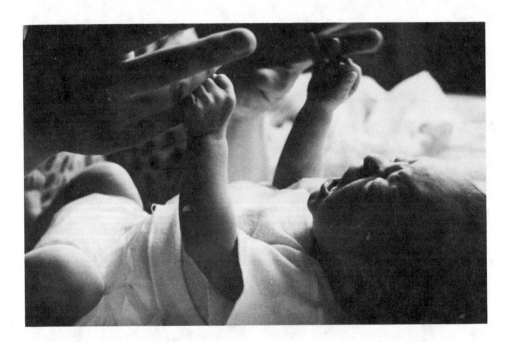

to a sitting position. Since your baby is not aware of holding on, be sure to give support with your other hand.

One common worry is that the baby will suffocate. This is not impossible, but your baby is born with a protective reflex to prevent this from happening. When lying face down, a baby's head will raise away from anything blocking the nose and mouth. At the very beginning this is a reflex, but within a few weeks your baby learns to control this ability, to lift the head on purpose for protection or to see more.

The smile is also a reflex at first. It is your baby's natural expression of pleasure and sometimes of discomfort.

Sudden or sharp noises cause the "startle" reflex. After a few experiences with a sharp sound, however, your baby will become accustomed to it and cease to startle. Music and other soft sounds may soothe your baby. From early on you can see your baby moving and smiling in response to the rhythms of your speech.

As you begin to enjoy and communicate with your newborn baby, you will begin to recognize and understand the signals and cues your baby uses to communicate needs, pleasures, and discomforts. Like adults, babies use gestures, expressions, and postures to let you know when they are pleased or displeased. Since they are not inhibited by social conventions, they readily show their feelings.

Signals and cues

Some ways your baby tries to involve you and win your attention are by widening the eyes, opening the hands, raising the head, assuming the feeding position, babbling, giggling, lip-smacking, smiling, gazing into your face, cycling arms and legs smoothly, and turning towards you. A baby uses these actions and noises to attract your attention, to let you know she or he likes your attention, and to prolong enjoyable situations.

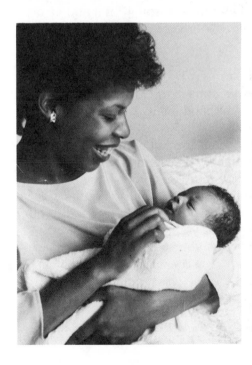
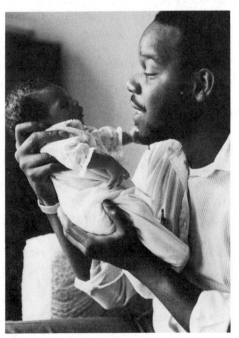

When your baby wants you to stop or slow down your play or talking, your baby may whimper, blink, clench eyes shut, look away; grimace, frown, pout, yawn; freeze into one position, kick, straighten the arms and legs, lower the head, join the hands or bring a hand to the ear, to the back of the neck, or to the mouth. If you do not respond to these signals, the baby often resorts to crying, whining, fussing, choking, vomiting, arching the back, pulling away, pushing away, or turning the head away. When you respond to your baby's initial, more subtle signs of distress, you both feel more comfortable. As babies and parents live and grow together, babies learn which cues to send and parents learn how best to respond to them. A unique give-and-take relationship develops and becomes increasingly "fine tuned" and supportive.

Often an uncomfortable or distressed baby resorts to self-comforting measures—moving hands to mouth, making sucking motions, fanning out fingers, sucking on fingers or fist, quieting and becoming still to pay attention to voices or faces, or changing position. If these measures fail, the baby will signal you for help. As parents and babies learn about each other they learn which consoling measures work best under which circumstances. Some babies respond to touching, swaddling, or having their hands gently held. Some babies calm when you hold them as you sit perfectly still. Other babies like to be held and walked about or rocked rhythmically and gently. Some babies like to be placed face down in a familiar crib and touched or patted. Other babies are soothed by a bit more feeding or sucking on a pacifier. Over time, through trial and error, you will discover the best ways to comfort your baby.*

Feeding signals   Most babies signal hunger by crying. Before crying, however, your baby may assume the "hunger posture"—lower arms held close to the abdomen and hands moving over the trunk, abdomen, and chest, or making a fist with palms toward the body.

When your baby begins to feel full, he or she will relax, often folding hands together, touching an ear with a hand, or lowering the arms to the sides with fingers extended. As satisfaction increases, your baby may stop sucking periodically for three-to-ten second intervals. These pauses will probably entice you to look at, stroke, rock, jiggle, talk to, or cuddle your baby who may at this time be more eager for your attention than for food. Indeed, the suck-pause pattern may be your baby's way of carrying on a conversation during feeding.

As your baby grows a little older, she or he will send you other signals to indicate when feeding time is over—shaking the head or turning

---

* For further information about signals and cues, see "Social Expressivity During the First Year of Life" by David Givens.

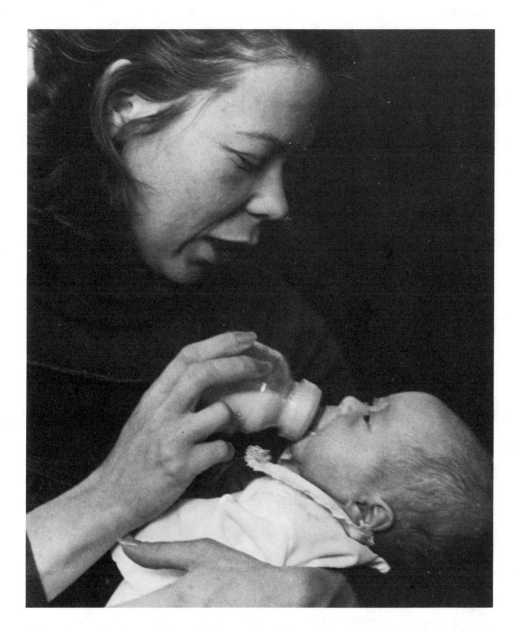

away from the breast, bottle, or spoon. If you do not get the message, your baby may arch the back, put a hand behind the head or ear, stick out the tongue making an "ugh" face, look away, pout, or beat with the hands. On the other hand, your baby may merely look away, then make eye contact with you when it's time for another suck or spoonful.*

* For a thorough guide to your baby's first three years of life, see *Good Beginnings* by Judith Evans and Ellen Ilfeld, available from LCPA and the High/Scope Press.

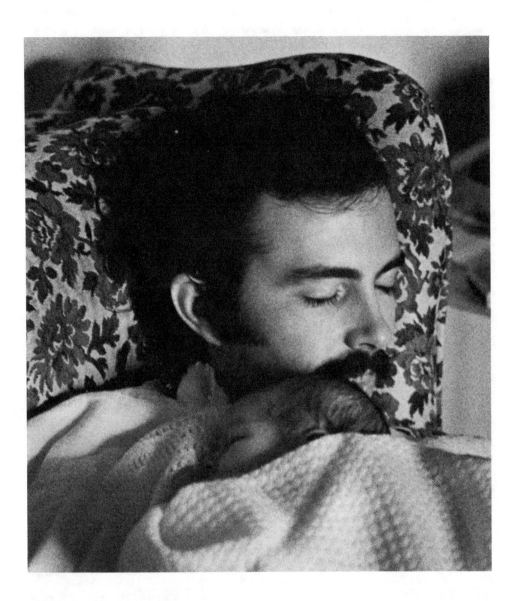

Growing together

Although it may seem like it at times, caring for your baby does not require magic. It does require patience, time, and commitment to a private, intimate relationship that is both demanding and rewarding. As you learn to know your baby's particular language of cues and signals and to appreciate your baby's marvelous strengths and abilities, you will enjoy and understand each other as you grow together.

Glossary

Abdomen The part of the body between the chest and the pelvis.

Amniocentesis A procedure whereby a sample of amniotic fluid is taken from the mother's uterus to diagnose certain congenital and hereditary abnormalities in the baby and to determine fetal lung maturity. A needle is inserted through the mother's abdominal wall into the amniotic sac. About half an ounce of amniotic fluid is withdrawn.

Amniotic fluid A clear, water-like fluid contained in the membranous sac (bag of waters) surrounding the baby in the uterus. It serves to support the baby, to permit the baby to move, to prevent heat loss, and to absorb shocks.

Amniotomy A method of inducing labor by rupturing the membranes. During a vaginal exam, the health care provider uses a sterile instrument to prick a small hole in the membranes. After this procedure, contractions are often closer together, longer lasting, and more intense.

Analgesics Drugs that help relieve pain without causing unconsciousness.

Anesthetic A drug used to induce loss of sensation and motor function with or without loss of consciousness.

Anterior position When the back of the baby's head faces the front (anterior) of the mother in the uterus.

Anus The outlet of the rectum, located directly behind the birth outlet (vagina).

Apgar score A quick and easy method of assessing a baby's heart rate, breathing, color, reflex response, and muscle tone. A nurse gives a baby an Apgar score twice, once at one minute after birth and again at five minutes after birth. A baby with a low score may need special observation and care.

Areola The pigmented area of the breast around the nipple.

Bloody show See Show.

Bonding A set of complex responses and behaviors through which babies and parents become familiar and committed to each other. Bonding or attachment is a gradual process that begins in the uterus and continues after birth as parents and babies meet, touch, and communicate.

Braxton-Hicks contractions Intermittent contractions of the uterus that are increasingly noticeable in late pregnancy as the uterus prepares itself for delivery.

Breech position A position in which the baby's feet or buttocks settle into the mother's pelvic basin so that during delivery the presenting part of the baby is the buttocks or the legs rather than the head.

Catheterization (urinary) The emptying of the bladder by insertion of a small, pliable tube through the urethra.

Centimeter The unit of measurement used to describe progress in dilatation. Used interchangeably with "fingers" (one finger equals two centimeters).

Cervix The narrow, necklike opening of the uterus.

Cesarean delivery Delivery of the baby through a surgical incision in the mother's abdominal wall and uterus rather than through the mother's vaginal canal.

Cesarean section See Cesarean delivery.

Chest breathing Keeping respirations high by expanding the rib cage when breathing—as opposed to abdominal breathing.

Coccyx The small, movable bone at the end of the spinal column. The tailbone.

Complete A term used to indicate complete dilatation of the cervix. A woman is said to be complete when her cervix is sufficiently dilated for the baby to pass through (usually ten centimeters, five fingers, or about four inches in diameter and 13 inches in circumference).

Contraction The tightening and shortening of the uterine muscles during labor, which causes effacement and dilatation of the cervix and contributes to the descent of the baby through the birth canal.

Crowning The appearance of the presenting part of the baby during the second stage of labor.

Diaphragm The muscular membrane separating the abdomen from the chest cavity. It contracts with each inspiration and relaxes with each expiration.

Dilatation The gradual expansion of the cervix until it is wide enough for the baby to fit through. Dilatation is measured by estimating the diameter of the opening cervix in centimeters or fingers.

Doptone An electrical instrument used to amplify the fetal heart tones.

DR A hospital term for delivery room.

Effacement The thinning of the cervix.

Effleurage A gentle, rhythmic, circular massage of the abdomen, back, or thighs. A comfort measure during labor.

Engagement When the baby's presenting part has positioned itself in the upper opening of the pelvis. This is the beginning position for the baby's passage through the pelvic structure. Sometimes called "lightening" or described by saying "the baby has dropped." Usually makes mother's breathing easier.

Engorgement The swelling of a woman's breasts three to five days after giving birth. Lasts several days and is caused by an increased blood and milk supply in the breast tissues.

Epidural space The space in the spinal column where an epidural anesthetic can be administered during labor or birth.

Episiotomy An incision made in the mother's perineum, between the vaginal opening and the anus, prior to delivery. It eases the baby's passage by widening the vaginal outlet.

Estriol A hormone found in the woman's urine during pregnancy. Estriol level is a simple, rapid, inexpensive method of determining various conditions of late pregnancy.

Fallopian tubes The two small tubes extending from either side of a woman's uterus to the left and right ovaries. When the ripened ovum is expelled from an ovary, it travels through one of the Fallopian tubes to the uterus.

False labor Regular or irregular contractions of the uterus strong enough to be interpreted as true labor, but not strong enough to dilate the cervix. Also called prodromal labor.

Fertilization The fusion of the sperm and ovum, normally occurring in the Fallopian tube. Conception.

Fetal heart tones (FHT) The baby's heartbeat through the mother's abdominal wall in the latter part of pregnancy (120-140 beats/minute).

Fetal monitor An electronic device used to continuously monitor and record uterine pressure and fetal heart rate. Internal fetal monitoring is possible when the woman's cervix is two to three centimeters dilated, the baby's presenting part is engaged in the pelvis, and the membranes have ruptured or can be ruptured safely. A small catheter is inserted through the cervix into the uterus to measure uterine pressure. A small wire is also attached to the baby's head. External fetal monitoring can occur at any time since recording is done using belts and sensors on the mother's abdomen.

Fetoscope An instrument used during labor to listen to the fetal heart rate.

Fetus A scientific term for the baby from the end of the third month of pregnancy until birth.

First stage of labor The period of labor when the cervix effaces and dilates to let the baby pass through. It is the longest part of labor. (90% of labor occurs during the first stage.) It ends when the cervix is dilated to ten centimeters.

Fontanelle A soft spot on the head of a newborn baby where the four bones of the skull have not yet grown together.

Fundus The top or upper portion of the uterus.

Induction Starting labor by medical intervention—stripping or rupturing the membranes or administering a contraction-stimulating hormone.

Intravenous To inject a sterile fluid into a vein to provide fluids, nutrition, or medication.

In utero Inside the uterus.

IV A hospital term for intravenous.

Labia The external folds around the opening of the vagina and urethra.

Let-down reflex The release of milk from the milk ducts sometimes described as a tingling sensation, a pins-and-needles feeling, or a sudden feeling of fullness in the breasts.

Lightening See Engagement.

Lochia The discharge of blood and mucus from the uterus after the birth of the baby. May continue several weeks and vary in amount.

Meconium Excrement in the fetal intestine.

Membranes The membranes or bag of waters that surround and protect the baby in the uterus.

Molding The shaping of the baby's head to adjust to the size and shape of the birth canal.

Mucous plug A plug of thick mucus that blocks the cervical canal during pregnancy.

Multipara A woman who has previously given birth. Abbreviation: M-2 or Multip.

Neuromuscular control The ability to make your muscles do what you want them to do. Synonymous with complete release, controlled release, controlled or active relaxation.

Occiput The back of the baby's head.

Ovaries The female reproductive glands where the ovum or egg develops prior to fertilization.

Ovulation The monthly release of a ripe ovum from an ovary.

Ovum The female egg cell.

Oxytocic drug A drug given to stimulate uterine contractions. Useful in starting labor, aiding labor, and stopping bleeding after delivery.

Pant-blow A series of light, shallow pants followed by a quick blow. May help control a premature urge to push in labor.

Patterned breathing Lamaze breathing patterns for labor and delivery designed to help a laboring woman relax, focus her concentration, and maintain an adequate supply of oxygen with a minimum expenditure of energy. See Slow chest-breathing, Shallow chest-breathing, Pant-blow.

Pelvic floor An interrelated muscle group forming support for the rectum, urethra, bladder, and internal reproductive organs.

Pelvis The bony ring joining the spine and legs. Its central opening forms the walls of the birth canal.

Perineum The external tissues surrounding and including the anus and vulva.

Pit drip A hospital term for an intravenous solution containing Pitocin, an oxytocic drug used to induce or enhance labor.

Placenta The vascular structure through which fetal nutrition, excretion, and respiration occur. Also called the "afterbirth."

Posterior position When the back of the baby's head faces the back (posterior) of the mother in the uterus.

Postpartum After giving birth.

Prenatal Before giving birth.

Primipara A woman who is having her first baby. Abbreviation: P or Primip.

Prodromal labor See False labor.

Psychoprophylaxis Using the mind to dull physical pain and to prevent the pain caused by psychological fear and body tension.

Relaxing breath A deep breath taken in through the nose and let out through the mouth at the beginning and end of every contraction. Used as a cue to release tension. Also called a "cleansing breath."

Retraction To pull back. In labor, when the uterine muscles shorten causing the cervix to draw back and open.

Rooming-in When a newborn baby stays with the mother in her hospital room rather than in the newborn nursery. Permits the mother to care for her baby and feed her baby on demand. The duration of the stay may vary.

Second stage of labor The period of labor when the baby passes from the uterus through the vagina and is born. Can last a few minutes or several hours.

Shallow chest-breathing A quick, active, one-second inspiration through the nose with the mouth closed, followed by a passive, one-second exhalation. Used as the active phase of labor progresses and slow chest-breathing is no longer effective for comfort and relaxation.

Show The reddish-colored mucus that sometimes indicates the onset of labor and that is gradually discharged during labor. Caused by the sloughing off of the protective mucous plug that seals the cervix during pregnancy.

Slow chest-breathing Breathing in through the nose for two seconds keeping the mouth closed but relaxed, and exhaling through the mouth for four seconds. Used during the early phase of labor when normal respiration is no longer adequate.

Sperm The male reproductive cell produced in the testes.

Sphincter muscle Ring-like muscle closing a natural opening. For example, the anal sphincter or the urethral sphincter.

Station During labor, the relationship of the baby's presenting part to the ischial bones on the mother's pelvis.

Sutures Absorbable stitches used to join the edges of an episiotomy incision and to repair uterine and abdominal incisions after a cesarean delivery.

Term The completed cycle of pregnancy. A woman near her due date is called "at term."

Third stage of labor The period of labor after the baby is born until the placenta is expelled. Lasts on the average from one to twenty minutes.

Toxemia A potentially serious condition of pregnant women characterized by swelling, elevated blood pressure, and protein in the urine. Varies from mild to severe.

Transition The end of the first stage of labor when the woman is dilated between seven and ten centimeters. The most active phase of labor.

Trial of labor The opportunity for a woman who may need a cesarean delivery to labor under close monitoring to see if vaginal delivery is possible.

Ultrasound A prenatal test in which sound waves are bounced off the fetus and placenta, producing a picture used to determine fetal age, number of babies, location of the placenta.

Urethra The tube that carries urine from the bladder to the outside of the body.

Uterus The muscular, pear-shaped, female reproductive organ in which the fetus develops for the nine months before birth. Also called the womb.

Vagina The birth canal. The curved, very elastic, five-or-six-inch-long passage-way from a woman's vulva to her cervix.

Vascular Composed of blood vessels.

VBAC An abbreviation for vaginal birth after cesarean. Many physicians now believe that 65% of all cesarean mothers can deliver vaginally in a subsequent pregnancy.

Vernix caseosa A protective, white, cheese-like material covering a newborn baby's skin. Seen in varying amounts.

Vertex Head down.

Vulva The external female genitalia. Commonly used to refer to the external lips or folds in front of the vaginal entrance.

References

Aguilera, Donna, and Janice Messick. *Crisis Intervention.* St. Louis: C. V. Mosby Co., 1974.

The American Journal of Maternal Nursing. September/October, 1976.

Bampton, Betty A., and Joan M. Mancini. "The Cesarean Section Patient Is a Mother, Too." *JOGN*, July/August, 1973, pp. 58-61

Barber, Hugh R. K., and Edward Graber. *Surgical Disease in Pregnancy.* Philadelphia: W. B. Saunders Co., 1974.

Blackburn, Susan. "Sleep and Awake States of the Newborn." *Early Parent-Infant Relationships.* White Plains, NY: March of Dimes Birth Defects Foundation.

Blackburn, Susan. "State-Related Behaviors and Individual Differences." *Early Parent-Infant Relationships.* White Plains, NY: March of Dimes Birth Defects Foundation.

Bing, Elisabeth, and Gerald Barad. *A Birth in the Family.* New York: Bantam Books, Inc., 1973.

Bonstein, Isidore. *Psychoprophylactic Preparation for Painless Childbirth.* New York: Grune and Stratton, Inc., 1958.

Boston Children's Medical Center. *Pregnancy, Birth and the Newborn Baby.* New York: Delacorte Press, 1972.

Boston Women's Health Book Collective. *Our Bodies, Ourselves.* New York: Simon and Schuster, 1972.

Bower, T. G. R. *A Primer of Infant Development.* San Francisco: W. H. Freeman and Company, 1977.

Bradley, Robert A. *Husband-Coached Childbirth.* New York: Harper and Row, 1974.

Brazelton, T. Berry. *Infants and Mothers: Differences in Development.* New York: Dell Publishing Co., Inc., 1969.

Brazelton, T. Berry. *Neonatal Behavior Assessment Scale.* Philadelphia: J. B. Lippincott, Co., 1973.

Brazelton, T. Berry. *On Becoming a Family: The Growth of Attachment.* New York: Dell Publishing Co., Inc., 1981.

Caplan, Frank, ed. *The First Twelve Months of Life.* New York: The Princeton Center for Infancy and Early Childhood, 1973.

Caplan, Gerald. *Principles of Preventive Psychiatry.* New York: Basic Books, Inc., 1964.

Carr, Rachel. "How to Relax All Day Long and Then Go to Sleep at Night." *Woman's Day,* October, 1974, pp. 94-95.

Chabon, Irwin. *Awake and Aware: Participating in Childbirth Through Psychoprophylaxis.* New York: Delacorte Press, 1966.

Clausen, Joy Princeton, and others. *Maternity Nursing Today.* New York: McGraw-Hill, 1973.

C/Sec, Inc. *Frankly Speaking.* Framingham, MA: C/Sec, Inc., 1978.

Davis, M. Edward, and Catherine E. Scheckler. *DeLee's Obstetrics for Nurses,* 16th ed. Philadelphia: W. B. Saunders Co., 1957.

DelliQuadri, Lyn, and Kati Brechenridge. *Mother Care: Helping Yourself Through the Emotional and Physical Transitions of New Motherhood.* Los Angeles: J. P. Tarcher, Inc., 1978.

Deutsch, Ronald M. *Key to Feminine Response in Marriage.* New York: Random House, 1968.

Donovan, Bonnie. *The Cesarean Birth Experience, Updated Version.* Boston: Beacon Press, 1978.

Engel, Edgar L., and Donna Z. Meilach. "The New Mother's Health." *Redbook's Young Mother*. New York: The Redbook Publishing Company, 1976.

Eriks, Jayne. "Infant Talk." In Kathryn Barnard, ed. *Nursing Child Assessment Training*, NCAST Series. Seattle: University of Washington Press.

Evans, Judith, and Ellen Ilfeld. *Good Beginnings: Parenting in the Early Years*. Ypsilanti, MI: High/Scope Press, 1982.

Ewy, Donna, and Roger Ewy. *Preparation for Childbirth*. New York: Signet, 1972.

Fitzpatrick, Elise, and others. *Maternity Nursing*, 12th ed. Philadelphia: J. B. Lippincott, 1971.

Flanagan, Geraldine L. *The First Nine Months of Life*. New York: Simon and Schuster, 1962.

Flowers, Charles E. *Obstetric Analgesia and Anesthesia*. New York: Harper and Row, 1967.

Gainer, Margaret Finnegan, and Patricia Madigan Van Bonn. "Two Factors Affecting the Cesarean Delivered Mother: Father's Presence at the Delivery and Postpartum Teaching." Research Report, University of Michigan, 1977.

Givens, David. "Social Expressivity During the First Year of Life." *Sign Language Studies*, Vol. 20, Fall, 1978, pp. 251-275.

Goodman, Louis, and Alfred Gilman, eds. *The Pharmacological Basis of Therapeutics*, 5th ed. New York: Macmillan, 1975.

Guttmacher, Alan F. *Pregnancy, Birth & Family Planning*. New York: Viking Press, Inc., 1973.

Hall, Robert E. *Nine Months' Reading: A Medical Guide for Pregnant Women*. New York: Bantam Books, Inc., 1965.

Hausknecht, Richard, and Joan Heilman. *Having a Cesarean Baby*. New York: E. P. Dutton, 1978.

Hawkins, Ida. "Natural Family Planning." *ICEA Sharing*, Spring, 1975, pp. 2-7.

Haynes, Una. *A Developmental Approach to Casefinding*. (U.S. Public Health Service Publication No. 2017.) Washington, DC: U.S. Government Printing Office, 1969.

Hazell, Lester Dessez. *Commonsense Childbirth*. New York: G. P. Putnam's Sons, 1969.

Heaney, Barbara Ann. *Suggested Parent-Child Activity List*. Grand Rapids, MI: Blodgett Memorial Hospital, 1981.

Hellman, Louis M., and others. *Williams Obstetrics*, 14th ed. New York: Meredith Corporation, 1971.

Holdcraft, Anita. "Obstetric Epidural Anesthesia." *Nursing Times*, November 6, 1975, pp. 1773-1775.

Hollinshead, W. Henry. *Textbook of Anatomy*, 2nd ed. New York: Harper and Row, 1967.

Hotchner, Tracy. *Pregnancy and Childbirth*. New York: Avon, 1979.

The International Childbirth Education Association. *The Childbearing Year*. Minneapolis: ICEA Publication Distribution Center, 1975.

Iorio, Josephine. *Childbirth Family-Centered Nursing*, 3rd ed. St. Louis: C. V. Mosby, 1975.

Klaus, Marshall H. *Maternal-Infant Bonding: The Impact of Early Separation or Loss on Family Development*. St. Louis: C. V. Mosby, 1976.

Krone, Carolyn. "Mental Health Needs of Women with High Risk Pregnancies." Unpublished manuscript, University of Michigan, 1976.

"Labor and Delivery Guide." New York: *American Baby Magazine*, 1977.

La Leche League International, Inc. "Breast-feeding After a Cesarean." (Information Sheet Number 80.) Franklin Park, IL: La Leche League, 1978.

Lavin, J. P., and others. "Vaginal Delivery in Patients with a Prior Cesarean Section." *Obstetrics and Gynecology*, Vol. 59, No. 2, February, 1982.

Maternity Center Association. *Birth Atlas,* 6th ed. New York: The Maternity Center Association, 1968.

McAllister, Roseanne G. "Obstetric Anesthesia—A Two Way Street." *JOGN,* January/February, 1976, pp. 9-13.

McCall, Robert B. *Infants.* Cambridge: Harvard University Press, 1979.

Mitchell, Kathleen, and Marty Nason, R.N. *Cesarean Birth, A Couples' Guide for Decision and Preparation.* San Francisco: Harbor Publishing, 1981.

Montagu, Ashley. *Life Before Birth.* New York: Signet, 1965.

Nilsson, Lennart, and others. *A Child Is Born: The Drama of Life Before Birth.* New York: Delacorte Press, 1965.

Nobel, Elizabeth. *Essential Exercises for the Childbearing Year.* Boston: Houghton Mifflin, 1976.

Norris, Catherine. "The Professional Nurse and Body Image." *Behavioral Concepts and Nursing Intervention.* Philadelphia: J. B. Lippincott Co., 1970.

Oxorn, Harry, and William R. Foote. *Human Labor and Birth,* 2nd ed. New York: Appleton-Century-Crofts, 1968.

Physicians' Desk Reference. Oradell, NJ: Medical Economics, Inc., 1977.

Planned Parenthood Federation of America, Inc. *Basics of Birth Control.* New York: The Planned Parenthood Federation, 1973.

Planned Parenthood Federation of America, Inc. *Questions and Answers About Intrauterine Devices (IUDs).* New York: The Planned Parenthood Federation, 1974.

Queenan, John T., ed. *A New Life: Pregnancy, Birth and Your Child's First Year.* London: The Van Nostrand Reinhold Co., 1979.

Reed, Constance. *Rapid Post Natal Figure Recovery.* Raritan, NJ: Ortho Pharmaceutical Corporation, 1967.

Riley, Harris, and Joan Berney. "Meeting the New Arrival: How to Arm Yourself for the Potential Battles Between Siblings." *American Baby Magazine,* April, 1982.

Rozdilsky, Mary Lou, and Barbara Banet. *What Now? A Handbook for New Parents.* New York: Charles Scribner's Sons, 1975.

Rubin, Reva. *Maternal-Child Nursing Journal.* Fall, 1975.

Russin, Ann Woolbert, and others. "Electronic Monitoring of the Fetus." *American Journal of Nursing.* July, 1974, pp. 1294-1299.

"Standards for Safer Baby Cribs." *Newsweek,* March 15, 1976, p. 72.

Stern, David. *The First Relationship: Mother and Infant.* Cambridge: Harvard University Press, 1977.

Sweet, Philothea T. "Prenatal Classes for Children." *Journal of Maternal Child Nursing.* March/April, 1979.

Taber, Clarence Wilbur. *Taber's Cyclopedic Medical Dictionary,* 10th ed. Philadelphia: F. A. Davis Co., 1965.

U.S. Department of H.E.W., Office of Child Development, Children's Bureau. *Prenatal Care.* Washington: U.S. Government Printing Office, 1962.

Vellay Pierre. *Childbirth Without Pain,* translated by Denise Lloyd. New York: E. P. Dutton, 1960.

Verny, Thomas, and John Kelly. *The Secret Life of the Unborn Child.* New York: Dell Publishing, Co., Inc., 1981.

Vest, Paul Joe, ed. *Nicholas and the Baby: A Study Guide.* Boulder, CO: Centre Productions, Inc., 1981.

Washtenaw County League for Planned Parenthood. *IUD.* Ann Arbor, MI: Planned Parenthood, 1975.

Washtenaw County League for Planned Parenthood. *Oral Contraceptives.* Ann Arbor, MI: Planned Parenthood, 1975.

Willson, J. Robert; Clayton T. Beecham; and Elise Reid Carrington. *Obstetrics and Gynecology,* 3rd ed. St. Louis: C. V. Mosby Co., 1966.

Wilson, Christine Coleman, and Wendy Roe Hovey. *Cesarean Childbirth, A Handbook for Parents.* Garden City, NY: Doubleday and Co., 1980.

Wright, Erna. *The New Childbirth.* New York: Pocket Books, Inc., 1971.

Young, Diony, and Charles Mahan. *Unnecessary Cesareans, Ways to Avoid Them.* Minneapolis, MN: International Childbirth Education Associaton, Inc., 1980.

Suggested Reading

The books on this list are not necessarily endorsed by the Lamaze Childbirth Preparation Association of Ann Arbor. They were selected to represent a wide range of options and viewpoints.

General guides to pregnancy and birth

Childbirth: A Manual for Pregnancy and Delivery by John S. Miller (New York: Atheneum, 1974). Includes Jacobson progressive relaxation routine.

Childbirth at Home by Marion Sousa (New York: Bantam Books, Inc., 1977). Well-researched book on why and how, with many references.

Commonsense Childbirth by Lester D. Hazell (New York: Putnam, 1969). A guide for mothers and fathers on giving birth the natural way.

A Guide for the Future Mother by L. M. Del Bo (Englewood Cliffs, NJ: Prentice-Hall, 1977). Thorough and sensitive medical guide including a large section on Lamaze.

Having a Baby by Eric Trimmer (New York: St. Martin Publishers, 1975). Diary and medical commentary with photos.

How to Be Happy Though Pregnant by Hyman Spotnitz, and Lucy Freeman (New York: Berkley Publishing, 1974).

Immaculate Deception: A New Look at Childbirth in America by Suzanne Arms (New York: Bantam Books, Inc., 1977). Critical examination of American obstetrical practice.

Joyous Childbirth: Manual for Conscious Natural Childbirth by E. J. Gold, and Cybele Gold (Berkeley, CA: And/Or Press, 1977). Preparation, experiences, and postpartum information.

Nine Months, One Day, One Year by Jean Marzollo (New York: Harper and Row, 1975). Facts and feelings about pregnancy, birth, and infancy—by and for parents.

Nine Months' Reading: A Medical Guide for Pregnant Women by Robert E. Hall (New York: Bantam Books, Inc., 1973). An annotated list of books for reading during pregnancy.

Pregnancy, Birth, and Family Planning by Alan Guttmacher (New York: Viking Press, 1973). Factual information to answer common questions.

Pregnancy, Birth, and the Newborn Baby by Boston Children's Medical Center (New York: Delacorte Press, 1972). Comprehensive guide by experts.

Preparing for Parenthood by Lee Salk (New York: Bantam Books, Inc., 1975). Understanding feelings to practicalities of life with a newborn baby.

The Relaxation Response by Herbert Benson (New York: Avon, 1975). Meditative technique.

Understanding Pregnancy and Childbirth by Sheldon H. Cherry (New York: Bantam Books, Inc., 1975). General guide with a section on Lamaze techniques.

Prepared childbirth: Principles and options

Natural childbirth methods

Childbirth Without Fear: The Original Approach to Natural Childbirth, 4th ed., by Grantly Dick-Read (New York: Harper and Row, 1972). The original Read method of "natural" childbirth.

Childbirth Without Fear: The Principles and Practice of Natural Childbirth, 2nd ed., by Grantly Dick-Read (New York: Harper and Row, 1970). Same book as above. Different edition with different title.

Methods of Childbirth: A Complete Guide to Childbirth Classes and the New Maternity Care by Constance A. Bean (New York: Doubleday, 1974). Objective comparisons of the various methods.

The Lamaze method

Awake and Aware: Participating in Childbirth Through Psychoprophylaxis by Irwin Chabon (New York: Dell Publishing Co., Inc., 1966). Lamaze history, theory, and practical guide.

The New Childbirth by Erna Wright (New York: Pocket Books, 1971). British interpretation of Lamaze.

Painless Childbirth: The Lamaze Method by Fernand Lamaze (New York: Pocket Books, 1972). Theory by the master.

Preparation for Childbirth by Donna Ewy, and Roger Ewy (Boulder, CO: Pruett, 1976). Textbook on Lamaze training.

Prepared Childbirth by Tarvez Tucker (New Canaan, CT: Tobey, 1975). Lamaze training with emphasis on conditioning theory and how the techniques affect awareness of pain.

Thank You, Dr. Lamaze by Marjorie Karmel (New York: Doubleday, 1965). One woman's experience with "painless" childbirth. Responsible for bringing Lamaze method to U.S.

What Every Husband Should Know About Having a Baby: The Psychoprophylactic Way by Jeannette L. Sasmor (Chicago: Nelson-Hall, 1972). Lamaze training emphasizing the husband's role.

Selecting health care for yourself

How to Choose and Use Your Doctor by Marvin S. Belsky, and Leonard Gross (New York: Arbor House, 1975). Lessons in assertiveness.

Maternal nutrition and fetal development

Nutrition

Nourishing Your Unborn Child: Nutrition and Natural Foods in Pregnancy by Phyllis Williams (Los Angeles: Nash Publishing Corp., 1974). Menus and recipes for pregnant and postpartum women.

What Every Pregnant Woman Should Know: The Truth About Diet and Drugs in Pregnancy by Gail Sforza Brewer, and Tom Brewer (New York: Random House, 1977). Sound nutrition explained. Includes a discussion of toxemia and its prevention.

Fetal development

Caring for Your Unborn Child by Ronald Gots, and Barbara Gots (Briarcliff Manor, New York: Stein and Day, 1977). Discussion of common environmental hazards to developing baby including tobacco, alcohol, and non-prescription drugs.

The Child Before Birth by Linda Ferrill Annis (Ithaca, NY: Cornell University Press, 1978). Fetal development and the influence of environmental factors. Summarizes recent scientific findings.

A Child Is Born: The Drama of Life Before Birth by Lennart Nilsson, and others (New York: Dell Publishing Co., Inc., 1966). Astonishing photos of baby's earliest development.

The First Nine Months of Life by Geraldine L. Flanagan (New York: Simon and Schuster, 1962). Prenatal development week by week in photos and text.

From Conception to Birth: The Drama of Life's Beginnings by Roberts Rugh, and others (New York: Harper and Row, 1971). Detailed, illustrated account of prenatal development, including genetics and environmental effects.

Is My Baby All Right? by Virginia Apgar, and Joan Beck (New York: Pocket Books, 1974). Causes and prevention of birth defects.

Life Before Birth by Ashley Montagu (New York: New American Library, 1964). How a mother can influence her baby's development.

Life Before Birth by Lennart Nilsson, and others (New York: Delacorte Press, 1976). Photos and up-to-date advice for parents.

Your Baby's Sex: Now You Can Choose by David Rorvik, and Landrum Shettles (New York: Bantam Books, Inc., 1971). Specific instructions for increasing your odds for preferred sex.

Understanding your changing body during pregnancy

Analysis of Human Sexual Response by Ruth Brecher, and Edward Brecher, eds. (New York: New American Library, 1966). Lay summary of Masters and Johnson plus others.

Making Love During Pregnancy by Elisabeth Bing, and Libby Colman (New York: Bantam Books, Inc., 1977). Effect of pregnancy on sex: facts and feelings.

Naturebirth: You, Your Body and Your Baby by Danaë Brook (New York: Pantheon, 1976). Encourages the pregnant woman to gain confidence for birth by tuning in to her own body.

Our Bodies, Ourselves by Boston Women's Health Book Collective (New York: Simon and Schuster, 1972). Biological and psychological functions.

Planning ahead for your baby

Breast feeding your baby

Breastfeeding After a Cesarean by La Leche League International, Inc. (Franklin Park, IL: La Leche League). Gives support and ideas for cesarean mothers who want to breast feed.

Breastfeeding and Natural Child Spacing: The Ecology of Natural Mothering by Sheila Kippley (New York: Penguin Books, Inc., 1975). Benefits of natural mothering.

The Complete Book of Breastfeeding by Marvin Eiger, and Sally Olds (New York: Bantam Books, Inc., 1973). Complete guide discussing solutions to possible problems.

Nursing Your Baby by Karen Pryor (New York: Pocket Books, Inc., 1973). Includes a week-by-week description of early infant life.

Please Breastfeed Your Baby by Alice Gerard (New York: New American Library, 1971). Common sense guide to breast feeding.

Preparation for Breastfeeding by Donna Ewy, and Roger Ewy (New York: Doubleday and Co., Inc., 1975). Complete guide to breast feeding.

The Tender Gift: Breast Feeding by Dana Raphael (Englewood Cliffs, NJ: Prentice-Hall, Inc., 1973). Emphasizes "mothering the mother" to ensure successful breast feeding.

The Womanly Art of Breastfeeding by Mary B. Carson, ed. (Franklin Park, IL: La Leche League International, 1963). Years of La Leche experience condensed for the nursing mother.

Outfitting your baby

Good Things for Babies: A Catalog and Sourcebook of Safety and Consumer Advice about Products Needed During the First 24 Months of Baby Life by Sandy Jones (Boston: Houghton Mifflin, 1976).

Guide to Buying for Babies by Consumer Reports Editors (New York: Warner Books, 1975). Brand name items rated for safety, value, and durability.

Preparing older children for a new family member

How Babies Are Made by Andrew Andry, and Steven Schepp (Alexandria, VA: Time-Life, 1968). Animal and human reproduction. Illustrated with paper sculptures.

How Was I Born? A Photographic Story of Reproduction and Birth for Children by Lennart Nilsson (New York: Delacorte Press, 1975). Good photographs.

A New Baby Is Coming to My House by Chihiro Iwasaki (New York: McGraw-Hill Book Co., 1970). Story of a child planning to welcome a new sibling.

On Mother's Lap by Ann H. Scott (New York: McGraw-Hill Book Co., 1972). Eskimo boy learns there's always room—even for a new baby. For pre-schoolers.

Where Did I Come From? by Peter Mayle (Secaucus, NJ: Lyle Stuart, Inc., 1973). Explicit, humorous cartoons.

Where Do Babies Come From? by Sheila Bewley, and Margaret Sheffiels (New York: Alfred A. Knopf, Inc., 1973). Explicit pastel paintings in an honest, but not a frightening presentation.

The Wonderful Story of How You Were Born by Sidonie M. Gruenberg (New York: Doubleday and Co., 1970). Designed for school-age children to read. Can also be read to younger children. Beautifully illustrated.

Preparing for labor and delivery

Essential Exercises for the Childbearing Year: A Guide to Health and Comfort Before and After Your Baby Is Born by Elizabeth Nobel (Boston: Houghton Mifflin, 1976). Prenatal and postnatal exercises.

Moving Through Pregnancy by Elisabeth Bing (New York: Bantam Books, Inc., 1975). Body mechanics, exercises, and "non-exercises" for the busy woman.

Prenatal Yoga and Natural Birth by Jeannine O. Medvin (Albion, CA: Freestone Publishing Co., 1974). Yoga principles applied to physical conditioning for childbirth. Includes photos of actual birth.

Labor and birth

Your childbirth partner

Husband-Coached Childbirth by Robert A. Bradley (New York: Harper and Row, 1973). Husband's supportive role during pregnancy and labor.

Variations in labor and birth

The Birth Primer, A Source Book of Traditional and Alternative Methods in Labor and Delivery by Rebecca Rowe

Parfitt (Philadelphia: Running Press, 1977). Comprehensive guide includes discussions of various methods for childbirth preparation and effects of labor medications.

The Cesarean Birth Experience by Bonnie Donovan (Boston: Beacon Press, 1978). Addresses a wide variety of issues regarding cesarean delivery and postpartum recovery. Includes some birth experiences.

Emergency Childbirth: A Manual by Gregory J. White (Danville, IL: Interstate Printers and Publishers, 1958). Police Training Foundation guide for the lay birth-assistant.

Frankly Speaking, 2nd ed., by C/Sec, Inc. (Framingham, MA: C/Sec, Inc., 1978). General information on cesarean delivery. Includes a section on vaginal delivery after a cesarean.

Having a Cesarean Baby by Richard Hausknecht, and Joan Rattner Heilman (New York: E. P. Dutton, 1978). Covers issues related to cesarean delivery. Some emphasis on how to plan for future deliveries.

Mothercare, Helping Yourself Through the Emotional and Physical Transitions of New Motherhood by Lyn DelliQuadri (Los Angeles: J. P. Tarcher, Inc., 1978). Overall guide to the adjustments one makes to new motherhood. Has a section on cesarean delivery.

What Now? A Handbook for New Parents by Mary Lou Rozdilsky, and Barbara Banet (New York: Charles Scribner and Sons, 1975). Guide for all new parents once home with their new baby. Has a special section for cesarean parents.

Birth experiences

Birth by Ceterine Milinaire (New York: Harmony, 1974). Interviews with parents, photos, hints, helpful information.

A Birth in the Family by Elisabeth Bing, and Gerald Barad (New York: Bantam Books, Inc., 1973). Photo story of Lamaze birth experience.

Birth Without Violence by Frederick LeBoyer (New York: Alfred A. Knopf, 1975). Poetic essay and photos on making birth a less stressful event for the baby.

The Experience of Childbirth by Sheila Kitzinger (New York: Penguin Books, 1972). Childbirth and parenting with focus on psychological aspects.

The Home Birth Book by Charlotte Ward, and others (Rockville, MD: Inscape Corp., 1976). Comments from all members of a home birth team.

The Pregnancy Notebook by Marcia C. Morton (New York: Bantam Books, Inc., 1972). A mother's notes.

Pregnancy: The Psychological Experience by Arthur D. Colman, and Libby Colman (New York: Bantam Books, Inc., 1977). Insights from a parent group discussion.

The Psychology of Childbirth by Aidan Macfarlane (Cambridge: Harvard University Press, 1977). Explores psychological impact of many aspects of birth on the mother and baby.

A Season to Be Born by Suzanne Arms, and John Arms (New York: Penguin Books, 1973). Photo-essay of pregnancy.

After your baby is born

Postpartum adjustments

The Cycles of Sex by Warren J. Gadpaille (New York: Charles Scribner and Sons, 1975). Discusses how the child from infancy to adolescence, effects parental psychosexual development.

Human Sexual Response by Masters and Johnson (Boston: Little, Brown and Co., 1966). Explains the hormonal effects on postpartum sexuality and the effects of breast feeding on sexual response.

Our Bodies, Ourselves by Boston Women's Health Book Collective (New York: Simon and Schuster, 1972). Explains the biological and psychological changes of the postpartum woman.

Sexuality and Man by Mary S. Calderone (New York: Charles Scribner and Sons, 1970). Discusses sexual relationships during pregnancy and postpartum changes that may occur.

What Now? A Handbook for New Parents by Mary Lou Rozdilsky, and Barbara Banet (New York: Charles Scribner's Sons, 1975). Suggests ways to improve postpartum intercourse and describes the father's postpartum feelings.

Contraception

The Complete Reference Book on Vasectomy by Michael Greenfield, and William M. Burrus (New York: Avon Books, 1973). Zero population growth orientation.

Contraception by Selig Neubardt (New York: Pocket Books, 1968). Brief but detailed encyclopedia of methods.

Natural Family Planning: The Ovulation Method by John J. Billings (Seattle: ICEA). Determining fertile period through cervical mucus changes.

Pregnancy, Birth, and Family Planning by Alan Guttmacher (New York: Viking Press, 1973). Factual information to answer common questions.

Vasectomy: Truth or Consequences by John J. Fried (New York: Saturday Review Press, 1972). Serious consideration of possible side effects.

Your newborn baby

Bonding

Maternal-Infant Bonding: The Impact of Early Separation or Loss on Family Development by Marshall H. Klaus, and John H. Kennell (St. Louis: Mosby, 1976). The importance of early contact for the development of a close mother-infant bond.

Newborn characteristics

Baby and Child Care by Benjamin Spock (New York: Pocket Books, Inc., 1976). Well-known, reliable guide for parents.

The First Twelve Months of Life: Your Baby's Growth Month by Month by Princeton Center for Infancy and Early Childhood, Frank Caplan, ed. (New York: Dunlap, 1973). Baby's development with discussion and many photos.

Good Beginnings: Parenting in the Early Years by Judith Evans, and Ellen Ilfeld (Ypsilanti, MI: High/Scope Press, 1982). The first section describes the characteristics of the newborn: Heads Up (0-1 month).

Infants and Mothers: Differences in Development by T. Berry Brazelton (New York: Dell Publishing Co., 1969). Follows the development of three different infants through their first year.

Reflexes, signals, and cues

"Engagement-disengagement Early Object Experiences" by Beatrice Beebe, and Daniel Stern. *Communicative Structures and Psychic Structures*, N. Freeman and S. Grand, eds. (New York: Plenum Press, 1977, pp. 35-55).

"The First Relationship: Infant and Mother" by Daniel Stern. *The Developing Child Series*. (Cambridge: Harvard Press, 1977). Examines the early social interactive process—the behavior of both the caregiver and the infant—as well as the structure, goals, and developmental functions of the process.

"The Origins of Reciprocity: The Early Mother-Infant Interaction" by T. Berry Brazelton, and others. In *The Effect of the Infant on Its Caregiver*, M. Lewis and L. Rosenblum, eds. (New York: John Wiley and Sons, 1974). Addresses the rhythmic quality of the infant's interaction with people and things. Measures the cyclic quality of attention and withdrawal; identifies non-verbal behaviors.

"Social Expressivity During the First Year of Life" by David Givens. *Sign Language Studies*, 20:251-274, 1978. Based on observations of the Nursing Child Assessment Project feeding and teaching tapes of babies at one, four, eight, and twelve months. Identifies specific non-verbal infant cues.

Parenting and child care

Child mental health

Child Behavior by Frances L. Ilg, and Louise B. Ames. Foreword by Arnold Gesell (Totowa, NJ: Barnes and Noble Inc., 1972). Reliable information on development based on findings from the Gesell Institute.

A Child's Mind by Muriel Beadle (New York: Doubleday and Co., 1971). Review of literature on child development to age five.

Every Child's Birthright: In Defense of Mothering by Selma Fraiberg (New York: Basic Books, 1977). How the human capacity to respond to others is determined by the relationship with the primary caregiver in infancy.

The Magic Years by Selma Fraiberg (New York: Charles Scribner and Sons, 1959). Commentary on the "interior life" of young children.

The Roots of Love by Helene S. Arnstein (New York: Bantam Books, Inc., 1977). How a baby learns to love.

Teaching the Child Under Six by James L. Hymes (Columbus, OH: Charles E. Merrill Publishing Co., 1974). What makes children tick from birth to age six.

Exercises for infants and children

The Baby Exercise Book: The First Fifteen Months by Janine Levy (New York: Pantheon, 1975). Developing baby's self-awareness through movement.

How to Keep Your Child Fit from Birth to Six by Bonnie Prudden (New York: Harper and Row, 1964). Exercises that hold the child's interest.

Touching: The Human Significance of the Skin by Ashley Montagu (New York: Harper and Row Publishers, Inc., 1971). Importance of the tactile experience.

Feeding infants and children

Complete Guide to Preparing Baby Food at Home by Sue Castle (New York: Doubleday and Co., 1973). Practical, easy to follow.

Feed Me, I'm Yours: A Recipe Book for Mothers by Vicki Lansky (Deephaven, MN: Meadowbrook Press, 1974). Emphasis on ease and nutrition.

Making Your Own Baby Food by James Turner (New York: Bantam Books, Inc., 1973). Alternatives to the standard diet for baby.

The Natural Baby Food Cookbook by Margaret E. Kenda, and Phyliss S. Williams (New York: Avon Books, 1973). Inexpensive, convenient foods for infants and toddlers.

The Organic Baby Food Book by Ann Thompson (New York: Trident Press, 1973). Over 200 recipes for do-it-yourself baby food. Includes seven-day menu plan.

Illness and accidents

Childhood Illness: A Common Sense Approach by Jack Schiller (Briarcliff Manor, NY: Stein and Day, 1972). When to call the doctor, what to do at home.

The Mother's and Father's Medical Encyclopedia by Virginia E. Pomerantz, and Dodie Schultz (Boston: Little, Brown, 1977). Complete health guide for parents.

Mothers' Medical Encyclopedia by Virginia E. Pomerantz, and Dodie Schultz (St. Louis: Formur International, 1975). References to all areas of child care.

A Sign of Relief: The First-Aid Handbook for Childhood Emergencies by Marvin I. Green (New York: Bantam, Books, Inc., 1977). Complete graphic instructions for dealing with emergencies.

Parenting guides

Bachelor Fatherhood by Michael McFadden (New York: Walker, 1974). How to raise and enjoy your children, as a single male parent.

Better Homes and Gardens Baby Book, Better Homes and Gardens, ed. (New York: Bantam Books, Inc., 1975). Practical, comprehensive guide to infant care.

Between Parent and Child by Haim Ginott (New York: Macmillan, 1965). Basic "childrenese." Sexist in part.

The Black Child by Phyllis Harrison-Ross, and Barbara Wyden (New York: Berkley Publishing Co., 1974). For all concerned with children in a multi-racial society.

Dare to Discipline by James Dobson (New York: Bantam Books, Inc., 1970). Control based on love and respect.

Dr. Turtle's Babies by William J. Turtle (New York: Popular Library, Inc., 1974). Guide organized around six areas of responsibility in child care.

Fathering by Maureen Green (New York: McGraw Hill, 1977). Recommends strong father role for security and happiness of children.

Father Power by Henry Biller, and Dennis Meredith (New York: Doubleday and Co., Inc., 1975). Encourages fathers to take a more active role in child rearing.

First Three Years of Life by Burton White (Englewood Cliffs, NJ: Prentice-Hall, Inc., 1975). Comprehensive guide with medical and emotional hints.

Good Beginnings by Judith Evans, and Ellen Ilfeld (Ypsilanti, MI: High/Scope Press, 1982). A thorough guide to the stages of growth and development from birth to age three. Includes age-appropriate activities.

The Great American Birth Rite by William Woolfolk (New York: Dial, 1975). A critical look at profit aspects and commercialism in childbirth and childrearing.

The Growth and Development of Mothers by Angela McBride (New York: Harper and Row, 1975). The "motherhood mystique"—how society's impossible expectations make mothers feel inadequate.

How to Bring Up a Child Without Spending a Fortune: The First Dollar-by-Dollar Guide to Beating the High Cost of Childrearing by Lee E. Benning (New York: Doubleday and Co., Inc., 1976). What to get and how.

How to Father by Fitzhugh Dodson (New York: New American Library, 1975). Focuses on fathering but relevant for mothers, too.

How to Parent by Fitzhugh Dodson (New York: New American Library, 1973). Art of parenting, by a psychologist.

How to Parent Alone: A Guide for Single Parents by Joan Bel Geddes (New York: Seabury, 1974). Tips for single parents.

How to Raise a Brighter Child by Joan Beck (New York: Trident Books, 1967). Learning in the important earliest years.

How to Raise a Human Being by Lee Salk, and Rita Kramer (Anderson, IN: Warner Paperback Library, 1973). How to promote your child's emotional health.

How to Raise Children at Home in Your Spare Time by Marvin J. Gersh (New York: Stein and Day, 1966). Practical, humorous approach to parenting.

Momma: The Sourcebook for Single Mothers by Karol Hope and Nancy Young (New York: New American Library, 1976). Resources and references.

Mothercraft by Margaretta Lundell (New York: Simon and Schuster, 1975). Collections of songs, games, recipes, and activities to bring joy to motherhood.

The Motherhood Book: Adventures in Pregnancy, Birth, and Being a Mother by Joan Wiener, and Joyce Glick (New York: Macmillan, 1974). Fresh look at young mothers.

The Mother Person by Virginia Barber, and Merrill M. Skaggs (New York: Schocken Books, 1977). Guidebook through the jungle of guilt, fear, and confusion of motherhood.

The Mother's Almanac by Marguerite Kelly, and Elia S. Parsons (New York: Doubleday and Co., Inc., 1975). Child care from the point of view of two mothers.

Now That You've Had Your Baby by Gideon G. Panter, and Shirley Motter Linde (New York: McKay, 1976). What to expect after your baby is born.

Parent Effectiveness Training: The Tested New Way to Raise Responsible Children by Thomas Gordon (New York: New American Library, 1975). By the originator of P.E.T.

Parenting: Principles and Politics of Parenthood by Sidney C. Callahan (New York: Penguin Books, 1975). Consciousness-raising for parents.

Peoplemaking by Virginia Satir (Palo Alto, CA: Science and Behavior Books, Inc., 1972). Concerned with family life and how humans are made.

P.E.T. in Action by Thomas Gordon (New York: Bantam Books, Inc., 1976). Basic P.E.T. techniques plus solutions from parents who use them.

Raising the Only Child by Murray Kappelman (New York: Dutton, 1975). Ideas for parents who plan to have one child.

Survival Handbook for Preschool Mothers by Helen Wheeler Smith (Chicago: Follett, 1977). Common sense advice on helping the infant develop self-esteem and confidence.

Toddlers and Parents: A Declaration of Independence by T. Berry Brazelton (New York: Delacorte Press, 1974). Survival and enjoyment of toddlers growing independently.

Toilet Training in Less Than a Day by Nathan Azrin, and Richard Foxx (New York: Simon and Schuster, 1974). A no-nonsense approach to toilet training.

Understanding Your Child from Birth to Three: A Guide to Your Child's Psychological Development by Joseph Church (New York: Pocket Books, 1976). Incomparable guide, practical, grounded in scientific research.

What Every Child Needs by Lillian Peairs, and Richard H. Peairs (New York: Harper and Row, 1974). Manual of practical child care.

What Every Child Would Like His Parents to Know by Lee Salk (Anderson, IN: Warner Paperback Library, 1973). Child care with the emphasis on preventative psychology.

What to Do When There's Nothing to Do by Elizabeth Gregg, and Boston Children's Medical Center Staff (New York: Dell Publishing Co., 1970). 601 ideas at minimum cost for ages 0-5.

Woman at Home by Arlene Rossen Cardozo (New York: Doubleday and Co., Inc., 1976). Support and ideas for the woman who chooses to make family her primary career.

Index